DUAL SENSORY IMPAIRMENT AND THE OLDER PERSON

Dr Annmaree Watharow and
Dr Moira Dunsmore

DUAL SENSORY
IMPAIRMENT AND
THE OLDER PERSON
An Invisible Epidemic?

The Disability Studies
Collection

Collection Editors
**Dr Damian Mellifont & Dr Jennifer
Smith-Merry**

LPp

First published in 2024 by Lived Places Publishing

British Library Cataloguing in Publication Data
A CIP record for this book is available from the British Library

ISBN: 9781915734358 (pbk)
ISBN: 9781915734372 (ePDF)
ISBN: 9781915734365 (ePUB)

Cover design by Fiachra McCarthy
Book design by Rachel Trolove of Twin Trail Design
Typeset by Newgen Publishing UK

Lived Places Publishing
Long Island
New York 11789

www.livedplacespublishing.com

Abstract

Is a decline in vision and hearing just a "fact of life" for people as we age?

Dual sensory impairment is an under-explored and little understood type of disability, but one which can have an enormous impact on those living with it and their partners, families, and carers. The number of people who are living with impairments to both sight and hearing is rapidly increasing as the global population ages, yet the challenges faced as a result are largely invisible. *The Third Sense* explores the experiences of older adults living with multiple or dual sensory loss, the social consequences, barriers, and stigma faced by people and their loved ones.

Drawn from the lived experience of both the authors and their research participants, this book is necessary and urgent reading for medical practitioners, clinicians, health workers, and social care providers in practice and training; higher education students of Disability Studies, Medicine and related courses, Social Work and related courses, Sociology, and Cultural Anthropology.

Key words

Hearing loss; vision loss; communication disability; ageing; inclusion; lived experience; sociology;social care; elder; gerontology.

Acknowledgements

Acknowledgement of country

We acknowledge and pay our deepest respects to the Gadigal people of the Eora Nation, the traditional custodians of the land on which we live, work and write.

We recognise the continued connection of First Nation peoples to the land on which we live, work and tell stories. We pay respect to Elders past, present and future and acknowledge that it always was, and always will be Aboriginal land.

Personal acknowledgements

ANNMAREE: As always, for any activity of research and writing, a dual sensory impaired person like myself is dependent on the kindness and skills of so many wonderful people. It is helpful if this help comes with good tea and cake.

Firstly, thank you to Moira Dunsmore, the greatest gift a co-author can give is to be there, to write, to critique and to think that a book writing book-camp in a five star hotel is a VERY good thing.

Thank you to Suzanne Wilding-Hart, for adding champagne to the necessaries of writing a book and supervising all the lovely accessibility assistants.

Accessibility is the fourth necessity of life (after air, water and cake) and thank you to my team of essential and lovely supports: Susannah Mcnally, Skye Wallace, Sophie Hague

The fifth element of good book-writing life is encouragement and advice, and we thank Dr. Julie Schneider, Roslyn Barnes, Dr. Riitta Lahtinen and Dr Isabelle Boisvert. A good life needs beautiful art. We can't thank Cathy Weiszman enough for the beautiful illustrations.

Thank you to David Parker for Reuben sandwiches and understanding when this took longer than expected. Damian Mellifont, you are a great editor and colleague, and we thank you for this. Finally, gratitude to my tolerant and patient family (Tony, Hannah-Rose, Oliver, Georgia and Eddie) who support me in all my endeavours no matter how hard.

MOIRA: Annmaree can be very persuasive! After finishing my PhD, my intent was to publish short articles for academic journals, and a book was definitely not on the horizon! However, our common ambition to advocate, draw much needed attention to dual sensory impairment in older persons and provide a 'toolbox' to health professionals based on the lived experiences of older persons with DSI, was too good an opportunity to miss.

The co-design and production of this book with Annmaree Watharow and the team (Damian Mellifont and David Parker) at Lived Place Publishing, has been a steep learning curve, but one filled with humour and creativity. I am very grateful to this 'web of support' for their encouragement, kindness and understanding as I navigated work-life-book balance, still a work in progress. Thank you, Dr. Julie Schneider (again), and Dr. Isabelle Boisvert, for your ongoing mentorship and academic guidance; thank you, Susannah McNally, Skye Wallace and Suzanne Wilding-Hart for making our meetings and writing sessions fun and welcoming, and of course, the tea and irresistible food.

To my family always, especially Ishbel and Mhairi, special thanks.

About this book

This book is written in a time where greater global attention is directed to ageing and the older person, not generally from a positive perspective. Much of the current narrative centers on burden: economic burden, social burden, demographic burden, caring burden, and of course, the burden to the health care system. While we acknowledge that ageing brings challenges to the older person, their family and social networks, we also know that changing the narrative around ageing in our society is critical to a more inclusive society, and a society that appreciates the wisdom, contribution and continued agency of older persons. Older people are very capable but may need *more* help to live happier, healthier and safer lives. That this help is not often forthcoming is an indictment of modern society. The lens of this book is one group of older people: those living with dual sensory impairments. This can be a bewildering and disabling experience, but it doesn't need to, nor should it be this way. With the globally rapidly ageing population and the consequent invisible epidemic of dual sensory impairment in older people in mind, we wrote this book.

The last few years of our research and writing has been marked by the ongoing COVID-19 pandemic. The pandemic has been cruel to many, and particularly for those with dual sensory impairment, young and old, who rely on physical touch, close proximity and lip-reading simply to communicate. Older adults, vulnerable to the effects of Covid-19, are well represented (too well represented) in current global and national mortality data. Maybe the pandemic has simply revealed pervasive societal attitudes that choose not to *'see'* or *'hear'* the more vulnerable older persons in our communities. In Australia, we have had two Royal Commissions that demonstrate ongoing systems of neglect; both highlight the invisibility and poor social recognition of older adults generally, and, specifically, those with a disability. Dual sensory impairment sits at the intersection of these two paradigms, as a poorly recognized disability, a 'feature' of older age with its pervasive impacts on health, wellbeing, quality of life, social interaction, functional ability and independence of older persons and their families. Perhaps the more relevant question is **why** are we not hearing their voices?

We, as co-authors, have come to realize through our studies, research and personal experiences that *'You're old, what do you expect?'* is the default for dismissing and minimizing conditions, symptoms and disabilities that ordinarily in a younger person would warrant care, support, even further investigations! Dual Sensory Impairment is one such condition. It is a poorly understood disability in older life that impacts a growing number of older adults in Australia and globally. In this book, we identify many of the structural challenges that exist in recognizing and diagnosing DSI, accessing support and rehabilitation, and providing care that is person-centered, acceptable and meaningful to the older person and their family. We know that dual sensory impairment has consequences for late-life independence, capacity for ageing in place and quality of life; as such, this compilation of research, lived experience narratives, and recommendations is designed to support health and social care students and professionals to address both the health ***and*** social aspects of dual sensory impairment.

This book is informed by, co-designed and inclusive of the narratives of older persons with DSI. We have designed this book to provide evidence in the form of peer reviewed literature, as well as (and most importantly), evidence from the lived experience of older persons with DSI, *and* their family carers. As an 'invisible' population, we have sought to 'render through writing' the facts, experiences and personal meaning of dual sensory impairment to older persons, but also to offer some recommendations based on research and evidence from a wide variety of sources.

The book is ideal for 'dipping in and out', as a resource to inform you, the health and social care student or professional, of the experiences of dual sensory impairment, and suggest reasons why social isolation, dependence and functional decline occur in older adults with dual sensory impairment. Importantly, we take a solution-based, capacity-building approach and provide recommendations that are person-centered, flexible and effective.

Contents

Learning objectives   xv

Chapter 1   Dual sensory impairment realities   1

Chapter 2   Understanding dual sensory impairment:
Definitions, prevalence, invisibility   17

Chapter 3   Dual sensory impairment: Health,
well-being, and security   37

Chapter 4   Seeing the unseen: Hearing the unheard:
Charles Bonnet syndrome and tinnitus   59

Chapter 5   The effort and art of caring   87

Chapter 6   The impact of DSI on building
and maintaining social networks   107

Chapter 7   Living better: Communication 1: Basics
for health and social care professionals/
practitioners   127

Chapter 8   Living better: Communication 2:
Social-haptic communication   151

Chapter 9   Living better: Communication 3:
Name signs, print on palm, fingerspelling,
and personalized systems   185

Chapter 10   Being prepared: Hospital admission and
emergency planning   207

Chapter 11   Living better with DSI: Integration of care:
             Putting it all together   **219**

Bibliography   **237**

Recommended further reading   **269**

Index   **273**

Learning objectives

By the end of this book, we hope you can:

Understand:

- The challenges of living with dual sensory impairment as an older person, from their perspective
- The prevalence of dual sensory impairment in older people
- The silent epidemic of our ageing populations means increasing dual sensory impairment, disability and multiple chronic and complex health issues
- The effort and art of caring for people with DSI
- How the presence of dual sensory impairment complicates life, health and wellbeing
- How social participation is impacted by dual sensory impairment, especially for older people
- The general risks to health, security and wellbeing posed by dual sensory impairment for older people
- The specific distress caused by visual hallucinations and how forewarning and reassurance can help
- The impact of dual sensory impairment on family carers, which includes both effort and the art of caring
- The wide range of simple and low-cost assistive devices to aid communication
- The everchanging and constantly evolving number of accessibility technologies that you will have to explore yourselves

- Climate disasters, pandemics and other emergencies mean we all need emergency plans
- The increased risk of hospital admissions in a climate of poor accommodation and recognition means we need to provide support to improve preparation.

Ask:

- Your patients, clients, constituents and customers what they need
- Your patients, clients, constituents and customers what their goals are
- Your patients, clients, constituents and customers how can you help
- Your patients, clients, customers what communication methods work best and when
- The carers of your patients, clients, constituents and customers what they need

Identify:

- Patients, clients, constituents and customers experience the complexities of dual sensory impairment
- People with dual sensory impairment in your work and their diverse communication needs
- Possible communication solutions
- Carer burden
- Capacity building with better communication, disaster planning and hospital preparedness

Provide:

- Support
- Understanding
- Care and communication
- Accessible formats
- Devices
- Aids
- Individual specific methods of communication
- Care, support and education for carers

Practice:

- Being part of a person with dual sensory impairments super team of supports
- Being inclusive
- "Walking the talk" with accessibility
- Upskilling: learning more
- Learning touch messaging and incorporating into your practice
- Asking about your patients, clients, constituents or customers goals and providing support to achieve those
- Including carers and families in care and communication
- Exhibiting kindness and patience in all that you do

Recognize:

- That this is a growing issue as people live longer, and it is the responsibility of all health care practitioners to provide quality, equitable care and communication to older people with dual sensory impairment.

In this book:

1. We use the acronym DSI widely in the book to refer to people with co-occurring hearing loss and low vision, that is, those living with dual sensory impairment.

2. We believe in the capability of older people, and we acknowledge societal responsibility to provide the support needed to live happier, healthier and safer lives both at home in the community, and in quality residential aged care. We have a long way to go to achieve this.

3. We know globally and nationally populations are rapidly ageing. We also know we are not prepared for the consequences of this.

4. Dual Sensory Impairment in older people sits at the intersection of both disability and ageing with little recognition, investment or body of lived experience testimonies.

5. We believe in a social relational framing of disability, in which disability can be complex and contingent, with many 'layers', of which ageing is but one.

6. We also value the epistemic approach of Miranda Fricker (2007) in which all our knowledge building on dual sensory impairment in older people is built upon and with, testimonies of lived experiences. This book, and our research endeavors, are founded on qualitative narrative inquiry from those who are the expert-knowers: those living with dual sensory impairment, and their family.

7. We believe in the scholar activism approach (Paradies, 2017), where it is not enough to build knowledge and increase awareness via academic publications. Our knowledge must translate into benefit for the community. This is our

output: a book for the present and future health and social care professionals to encourage and guide approaches to their work with older people with DSI, with greater understanding, awareness and skills to help harness the capabilities of older people with Dual Sensory Impairment. This means society committing human support, accessibility technology and funding resources specifically for older people, their families and carers generally, and those with DSI specifically.

8.   Our next book adventure will involve the creation of a consumer handbook for those living with DSI, and their carers and families, to use as a text, a reference and a tool to support their journeys with dual sensory impairment.

1
Dual sensory impairment realities

Introduction

Dual sensory impairment (DSI), the combination of hearing loss and low vision, affects our lives in so many insidious, often invisible ways. We embarrass ourselves in company, knock over champagne glasses in restaurants, fall off unseen curbs. We struggle to work out what is going on around us. It is harder too, because our families don't always understand and our healthcare professionals don't recognize or acknowledge our DSI or, are too busy to provide needed information and support. And where is The Society for People Who Don't See Too Good or Hear Very Well? While there are services for people with deafblindness, most of us think DSI is all part of growing old.

The following accounts suggest what it's like to live with DSI, or to live with someone who has it. These experiences are about living with little recognition and social support generally. In fact, when we are supported with good information and quality communication, we are enormously capable human beings. In this chapter, we present personal experiences and verbatim testimonies from the authors, research participants, and their family members over one morning, afternoon, evening, and night—24 hours in the life of DSI. We thank Eva, Seraphina, Justine, Nina, Loretta, Francine, Nicole, Leah, Christine, Violetta, Gladys, Mabel, Sara, Daisy, Phillip, Victor, Loraine, Alan, Nelson, and Roy, for their words.

One day (and night) in the life of DSI

Morning

Mornings can be difficult for those living with DSI; they can be busy with getting ready for the day's appointments and activities. Eva has age-related hearing loss and diabetic retinopathy; she wakes around seven in the morning, beginning her day with a variety of communication woes, "I don't hear the alarm anymore so Phillip [Eva's partner] wakes me. Sometimes the day starts when he asks me something and I don't hear, so he yells at me, and I get all upset. It isn't even earth-shattering information he is after; mostly: 'Do I want a cup of tea?'. Then we snarl at each other for a while. It's not a good way to start the day. While this is going on, Phillip sorts out my tablets because I'm not allowed to anymore; I once spent a whole week taking antihistamines instead of important blood pressure stuff. They were the same size and shape".

Seraphina is aging with DSI, she has congenital blindness but acquired hearing loss in older age. She has fallen off an unseen curb and is now in hospital. The doctors are on their morning ward rounds. She observes, "Staff need to let me know they are there and give me time to put on my hearing aids. Doctors come on ward rounds and stand at the bottom of the bed, talking to each other and not to the patient in the bed. They mumble. No one takes the time to help me with what I need, so, I don't know what is going on".

Social activities can be arduous. Justine is invited out this morning, but she is looking for an excuse to decline, any excuse will do. She has age-related hearing loss and age-related macular degeneration and laments, "I don't particularly want to mix with people. Too hard. Too hard because they can't understand".

Mixing in crowds, at parties, and even among family and friends is difficult. Justine feels she has lost the art of good manners and conversation: "It's so embarrassing. They've said hello to me, and I think, 'Gosh who is it?'". Daisy too, has been living with aged-related hearing loss and macular degeneration for over 15 years, and like Justine, has progressively been disengaging from social activities, despite her daughter (and family carer) encouraging her to keep up with friends, hobbies, and clubs. She describes feeling embarrassed at her lack of ability to follow conversations and tells us: "I keep away from people. I'm all right one to one but I don't like socializing anymore because I can't keep in the conversation. I can't hear it".

There are major challenges associated with living in residential aged care aka nursing homes. These are not necessarily a haven for people with DSI. Eva worries if anything happens to Phillip, "I have no option but to go into a home". Victor says, "Family don't want us living with them when we have multiple disabilities". Victor has bilateral optic atrophy and hearing loss from occupational noise exposure. He wears hearing aids and loves it when others don't realize he is also blind. His wife Mabel has DSI as well as numerous other health conditions and is often in hospital. Since their families did not want to live with them, they moved into a "home" where there's no accommodation for a married couple, so Victor and Mabel have rooms 25 meters apart in the facility.

Victor says, "It's a bit like living on Mars since Covid, with all the gear, masks, shields, and gowns. Sometimes in an outbreak we are just stuck in our rooms for days, weeks, and even months, no one looking in or helping or anything". Victor compensates by supporting other residents with advocacy and supervision, "I'm the only one here able to do things. The rest are all too sick or too old to do anything". Victor and Mabel describe management as neglectful, "Everyone here is old and has disabilities…It is isolating…I've found three people dead here—I've got it going that if you haven't seen your neighbor…we need to know about it".

Alan is also in a "home": his daughter, Gladys, has come to visit this morning and she is frustrated that he doesn't have his hearing aids in…again. Alan has Alzheimer's disease, as well as DSI from his time in the army. He is comfortable wearing hearing aids, unusual for this older male demographic: "The catch is", says Gladys, "someone has to put them in, as he doesn't remember. And you know, when they do remember, the batteries are usually dead". She continues, "I am convinced that the staff here, lovely as they are, believe that there is no point putting them in when he has dementia. But really, he needs all the information he can get, however he can get it, to make whatever sense of whatever he can. It is more important now than before. My mum used to spend a lot of time orienting him and supporting his social conversations, but when she died that all stopped. We had thought that being here, this support would continue. We were wrong".

There's a lack of communication partners in "homes". Audrey describes what this means for her, "A few staff fingerspell or write on my palm or my arm. They will use a rubbing-out motion when a mistake has been made…. But a lot of them don't speak good English and so they can't spell. So, I don't understand what they are saying a lot of the time…. It gets lonely…I wait and wait and wait for someone to help me know what is going on".

Going to the doctor is particularly difficult. Loretta has Meniere's disease and retinal vascular disease; she has an appointment with her GP this morning. She struggles with doctors and nurses' voices—male voices, accents, and doctors using computers and not facing her. Loretta says that at the medical center and in the hospital, staff talk to each other and exclude her. She says, "They avoid you rather than communicate with you, and the GP is always hurrying me up, he decides what is important to cover and has no time to talk about the difficulties I am having with ordinary life things".

Today she frets, "I do hope he isn't looking at his computer instead of me…so hard to lipread…I always get stressed here and at the outpatients because I can never hear my name being called…. And Covid has just made things so much worse. Those masks and plastic face covering things. Before I could work out enough words to understand what people were talking about generally. Now I can't, so I just say yes and hope that's the right thing to say".

Francine agrees, "It's terrible, especially if I haven't got my husband to be my ears and eyes…. I wonder what people do when they don't have someone to help them? …. The blinder I get, the more I fall and if my husband isn't there, I feel like I'm in panic mode because I don't know what to do, I don't know what's happening around me. I really need someone by my side".

Loraine says life with a moderate hearing loss and light perception-only vision is "complicated", especially when interacting with healthcare. Despite Loraine being very ill for the first few days of her hospital stay, she had to continually educate healthcare professionals and carers. "What I find the most difficult— you must explain to every single nurse and every single doctor that you couldn't see properly, and you couldn't hear properly. I can't see the way to the bathroom. I can't see the buzzer; so, I can't find the buzzer to ask for help with going to the bathroom. When I finally found it, no one answered the call for help… other patients in nearby beds screamed out for the nurse. The next occasion I need the bathroom, I buzz, the nurse says, 'Oh, for God's sake, can't you wait?' Afterwards, I don't press the buzzer anymore because I am a nuisance…I am in tears".

Eva's husband is out, and she's expecting a delivery. Eva hates the doorbell ringing. "I can often hear the doorbell, but not always. I get so worked up when one of the kids says I've sent you a parcel and it's arriving today. I then must concentrate really carefully all day to make sure I don't miss it. Sometimes, I imagine the doorbell ringing and rush to answer and no one is there. Sometimes, someone I can't see or identify is on the doorstep and I have no idea what they want. I've got a little mantra now: 'Parcel? Do I need to sign?' Otherwise, I send them away and tell them to come back when I know Phillip will be home. Once I sent the police away like that".

Regular social events can be onerous; church on a Sunday morning should be a social highlight of the week, instead, Nicole says, "We go with 15 or 16 of us on Sunday morning—I've really debated about dipping out. My brother and sister-in-law go to church, and they sort of keep insisting that I go—but the noise, the surround[ings] with my hearing aids…I don't join in the conversation".

Afternoon

Afternoons with DSI can be tricky. Concentrating all morning may mean not much left in the tank for the afternoon. Nelson has age-related macular degeneration and age-related hearing loss. He says having DSI is "like driving into fog at night". He eats lunch with his granddaughter, Sara, who is now going to show him how to bank online. Nelson describes his experiences afterwards, "Honestly, young kids these days are just so fast, moving the mouse, click here, click there, the pages just whizz by. I'm too embarrassed to ask her to slow down, I just can't look at the laptop and listen to her explaining things at the same time". There is so much work in processing new information and learning new things takes so much longer.

There is hard work in socializing, sometimes too hard. Roy and Leah have always been socially active together; Leah has DSI and despite Roy planning many shared activities, most are declined by Leah. Roy relates, "I've been trying to get us to go for a picnic up the Hawkesbury or something and I can have a fish and Leah can sit there and listen to her book, in the park, just to get out.

That hasn't happened yet. I've even bought two folding chairs; they haven't come out the package yet and that's been a couple of years". Leah replies, "I am doing less because I can't be bothered".

Little things have a big impact. Victor's batteries have run out, so he needs to change them before heading out for afternoon visiting to see his wife in hospital, "And it is such a palaver, when will hearing aid makers develop ones that older people can actually use?" He wonders, "Hearing aids are hard to use…very hard, small buttons…batteries are difficult to change…I have to get someone to help tear the sticky paper off the back [of the battery]".

Loretta talks about trying to get some solutions for her worsening DSI, as she ages and how frustrating it is to know solutions are available; however, "Friends and family won't learn tactile language [so even if I learn] I won't be able to communicate with them".

Christine is at the ophthalmologist having been diagnosed with age-related macular degeneration, one of the commonest causes of low vision in older people. She feels the diagnosis is poorly explained and the doctor doesn't understand the impact of the low vison in combination with her aged-related hearing loss. She comments, "No. The ophthalmologist didn't explain at all. He simply asked me, 'Would you like to go to have counseling?' I didn't even know what counseling was. He told me, 'You will never go blind. Because your peripherals are so good'. So, he said, 'Just be grateful for that'".

Violetta would like to change her GP, as the present one who comes to her aged-care facility doesn't spend enough time with her, or use a communication method that works, or address the complex multiple disabilities she lives with. But staff say that her guardian must agree before this can happen. However, the guardian, a geographically remote relative, comes to visit only once or twice a year to attend a family meeting. Violetta says, "I am not invited to speak on any reviews of my care", so has no voice or agency to change her situation.

In the early afternoon, Leah visits the local bank. She has always done the family financials and is hanging onto this activity for as long as she can. She tells us, "I did everything—well, now I barely can, I can't read them, but they're used to me at the bank, they point and show me where to sign, God knows what I'm signing half the time. I can't write a check, but I have someone write it for me and I must always sign it, I won't let my husband, Roy sign it, just always me. Oh yeah, I'm hanging onto that".

Eva and Phillip go to see a popular exhibition of Impressionist paintings: Van Gogh Alive Interactive. Here, the paintings are shown digitally in very large format on the walls of the Convention Center. Phillip hopes that this will allow Eva to get some joy back from the art she used to love. As they walk, Phillip explains what they are seeing, so that Eva can make sense of the details she can see only at the periphery of the artworks. Phillip ducks off to the loo, a few minutes later Eva sees him again and walks over and puts her arm around him: "There you are, dear man". Only, it is not Phillip. A few seconds pass and the real Phillip returns asking, "What are you doing over here?"

Loretta is trying to buy her son a birthday present, "I would like to surprise him and his wife with a weekend away, but I can't organize things on the phone anymore because I can't hear, or buy online as the print is too small, and if I email, they say go online. I need to ask for help doing any shopping or booking things and it's all I do these days is ask for help. I work hard at not just giving up on it all. But it's very hard. And then someone will say, 'Loretta, you need to make more of an effort with things'. I really don't think people understand what it is like".

Justine and her daughter Nina are discussing etiquette and whether the expectation of reciprocity still exists. Nina says, "Mum feels bad. Mum says, 'They've invited me to their house, but I can't invite them back because it's too hard to make a cup of tea' but I sort of think people probably don't care, but that's the way we grew up that you always return the invitations". Justine replies, "It's not that I don't or wouldn't love to have people here, but of course you've got to have a cup of tea and a bickie, and I'll probably scald myself".

It's a bridge day for Nicole; she still goes even though she notes that fewer people are engaging with her. She says "Well, I go and sit, and I shuffle cards and I've noticed that I haven't got the people who will come by and say 'Hello' now, or 'How was the weekend?' or something. I just notice that it's a bit antisocial now because you can't hear that much….

Evening

Evenings are complicated times for many who live with DSI: fatigue, poorer concentration, less light, less motivation to engage. "Evening visiting is between three and eight pm at the hospital" says Victor. He goes to visit his wife, catching the lift. "I wish there were talking elevators in hospitals saying, 'Going up. First floor: Ward One North, Ward One South, Physiotherapy Department'". Mabel has been in hospital for a week already and Victor has had to learn the route to her room by heart: "No point asking anyone, they just point and say follow the yellow line and turn left at the fourth bay. So, me and my white stick just tap, tap our way along and hope for the best". This time, however, he finds Mabel's bed easily and sits down with a sigh, reaches for her hand asking, "How are you going, Darling?" Only it isn't Mabel. "You're not my wife!" Victor says. She's been moved (again).

Living with DSI in residential aged care is troubling. Seraphina calls it "aged-no-care", Victor calls it "neglectful", and Violeta says, "I hate my nursing home". For people with DSI "aged-no-care" is tough as they usually don't have a communication partner. Audrey observes, "In all the years I have been here, only two people have bothered to try and work out how to communicate better with me".

Evening is the time when staff are more likely to use restrictive practices of sedation or restraint to "manage" people with DSI. Violeta describes forcible medication, "The staff push my chin down and shove medicine in…when I can take it perfectly well if they put it in my palm". Night sedation is common in nursing homes even when residents don't want this. Violeta says, "Staff don't want me waking up and being difficult, so they sedate me which makes me sleepy during the day too".

For those living at home, social activities require significant effort. For example, going out for dinner is exhausting (even with hearing aids) because of the cacophony, but without hearing aids, there are only snatches of words. Leah detests it: "I hate it when I have other people at the table and we go out to dinner in a group of eight, I loathe it, you know because I swear blind, I can't hear as well because I can't see the faces, and expressions mean a lot, so yeah, I don't like that".

Francine lives at home and has gone out locally with some new friends; one of them laughs at her (snidely Francine suspects). She says, "He kept on pointing out every wobble and misstep I made. 'Been on the booze. Can't hold ya liquor. You're a bit of a lush, love'…awful, awful things. It was very distressing and when I asked him to stop, he said I didn't have a sense of humor. I couldn't take a bit of ribbing. I never went out with that group again".

Eva is out (reluctantly) with her close friend. Her friend tells her, "You have two different shoes on tonight! I'll read you the menu shall I? I'll leave out all the things I know you don't like as it's an exceedingly long menu!" Eva finds herself talking continuously as the restaurant is too noisy for her to understand conversations with the waiter and her friend. She suggests to her friend, "You pick dinner" as understanding the lengthy read out menu is difficult. When the meal comes, Eva is making a gesture and knocks over the wine glass.

For others with DSI, the evening is a time of waiting, and of feeling isolated; they may be inclined to participate socially but social, emotional, and physical barriers prevent them, as Justine says, "Everybody else is doing something and I'm sitting there waiting, so I go to bed, it's warm, it's safe".

Overnight

Night-time is dark time, time when there are fewer resources to help those with DSI work out where we are and what's happening.

Violeta is in hospital and wards off a nurse's hands. The nurse hasn't bothered to explain why she needs to touch Violeta and the touch is unwanted. Violeta says, "I don't like people touching my body all over without letting me know what they're intending to do….Someone tries, I think, to put in a new drip, but I bat their hands away".

"In hospital, you have to wait all the time" Violeta says. "I don't like waiting" she says, "I have to wait for the nurse, and I have to wait for the toilet. Sometimes, I have to wait so long that I wet myself. I'm in the too-hard basket. They don't know how to support me and, therefore, they just neglect me. And so, I am oblivious to what is going on".

Loretta says, "It is all very vexing as you want to be conscious of energy usage, but really I have got to have the hall light and bathroom light on all night as I am frightened of having a fall".

DSI is about loss. Eva has some residual vison, but it is not enough to read a conventional book: "I used to love reading, especially whodunits and historical fiction. If I woke up in the night, I would just grab my book and read myself to sleep again, or not! I really miss that…that's what I notice about the combination of hearing and sight loss is that it is all about loss. Loss of movies. Loss of theater. Loss of parties. Loss of reading. Loss of connection to old friends. Loss of ability to make new ones. Loss of independence. Loss. Loss. Loss. They've all gone".

Conclusion

This introductory chapter gives you, the reader, some insight into the day-to-day difficulties and frustrations experienced by those with DSI, and, in many cases, their families and carers. We also highlight here the many examples of ableism in action for those with DSI. Perhaps it makes you consider why older adults with DSI become socially isolated and reluctant to engage? The reality is the effort involved is immense and unremitting. We understand that social participation is considered an important issue for older adults; there is widespread recognition of the relationship between reduced social participation, social isolation, health status, and mortality. DSI, as described here, impacts not only the self but the partner, close family members, friends, friendship groups, and social or special interest networks. Yet knowledge of the level and type of support required to optimize social participation, health, and wellbeing for those with DSI is remains poor.

The invisibility of DSI also means that public knowledge is insufficient to support and understand not just those with DSI but what their friends and relatives are going through.

Another prominent feature of all these testimonies is that society, health and aged-care policy, health and aged-care institutions, and health and aged-care professionals are not doing enough to support older people to navigate their DSI, and in many cases additional multiple disabilities and chronic conditions. Fear of the future is rightly common for those living with DSI. Eva wonders about the lack of insight: "If poor hearing and sight are so common in older folk, how is it that aged-care services aren't equipping themselves to be supportive and communicate with us? I've seen the failures in nursing homes, in hospitals visiting friends and family, and I've experienced the disinclination to assist us in banks and shops. Frankly, I'm frightened to get any older, any deafer, and any blinder".

This book aims to bridge the gulf in knowledge about and around DSI. In Chapter two, we begin by defining what DSI is, presenting local and international data (and gaps in our knowledge), and then examining the invisibility of DSI.

2

Understanding dual sensory impairment

Definitions, prevalence, invisibility

Introduction

There are many different terminologies in use to describe the co-occurrence of hearing loss and vision loss. Some examples include deafblindness, dual sensory impairment (DSI), dual sensory loss, and multisensory impairment. Some people may use variations on the first impairment, e.g., blind with hearing loss or deaf with low vision. For many older people, no term is used, just an acceptance that not seeing too good and not hearing too well must be a "normal" part of aging. Researchers and professionals may use different terminologies to those actually living with co-occurring hearing and vision loss. Researchers and disabled people's organizations (DPO) may prefer to use deafblindness, rehabilitation providers working with older people may use DSI, while those working with children may use deafblindness.

And then there is the linguistic conundrum: identity-first versus person-first naming, as in for example, deafblind person or person living with DSI. Interestingly, the move for media reportage generally in disability has been from identity-first to person-first (Bednarek, Potts and Watharow, 2023) and likewise in government policy and practice in Australia. Yet among individuals living with disability, we see that identity-first language remains strong (Sharif et al., 2022). This reminds us all to ASK individuals and the DPO that we work with, what their preferred descriptor is.

In this work, we will use person-first language, e.g., person with a DSI or person living with a DSI. Where the first author and many of the contributors identify otherwise (e.g., as a deafblind person), we will use that preferred descriptor. As mentioned in the Introduction to this book, we will use hearing loss, d/Deafness, hard of hearing, and hearing impairment interchangeably for that single sense, and vision loss, vision impairment, or low vision for that sense. Blindness is also used to refer to more severe vision loss. Commonly however, we will use hearing loss and low vision for single sensory loss and DSI for the combination. This reflects consumer and/or DPO usage. Unlike the United Kingdom and the European Union, Australia does **not** recognize DSI or deafblindness as a unique and distinct disability. And this has a direct impact on perpetuating the prevailing lack of awareness and integrated service provision as well as a lack of accepted systemic terminology/ies.

Dual sensory impairment (DSI)

DSI describes the concurrent impairment or loss of both vision and hearing senses, which can occur across the lifespan but is increasingly prevalent in older adults (Dammeyer, 2014). We focus here on older adults with DSI who are poorly understood by existing research and poorly supported by existing services and policies. A very small percentage of older adults with DSI are aging **with** DSI, the vast majority (over 99 percent) are aging **into** DSI. For more on the particularities of aging with DSI, see Simcock and Castle, 2016, Simcock et al. 2023.

DSI is the umbrella term we will therefore use to describe the spectrum of combined vision and hearing loss in older adults, in which access to information, communication, as well as orientation and mobility are compromised. Both listening and speechreading communication are impacted, and hence, the capacity to interact socially is weakened (Heine and Browning, 2002, 2004). Challenges to communication impact the ability of older adults with DSI to participate meaningfully and engage in everyday functional activities (Brennan and Bally, 2007; Dammeyer, 2014; Jaiswal et al., 2018, 2020; Simcock and Wittich, 2019). The synergistic effects of combined vision and hearing losses, and reduced capacity to compensate one sensory loss with another, positions DSI as a unique and complex disability in its own right (World Federation of the Deafblind [WFDB], 2018) and as the "third sensory loss" (Simock, 2017). Many researchers, DPO, legislators, and service providers use an unhyphenated term "deafblind" to represent both the distinct disability status and the lack of ability of either sense to compensate for the other (Nordic Centre for Welfare and Social Issues, n.d.). This book acknowledges the wide use of "deafblind" in support and research but notes that none of the participants aging into DSI in our own work and worlds use the term "deafblind" to describe themselves (Dunsmore, 2022; Watharow, 2021). See Wittich et al. (2013) for a close examination of these contentions.

Distinct disability

Just over one third of 50 countries surveyed by the World Federation of the Deafblind (2018) recognized deafblindness–DSI as a unique and distinct disability. This limits understanding of DSI as a global disability. Without such recognition, people living with DSI, their carers and families, and the DPO that serve them don't have seats at the tables of protectors, legislators, policy makers, professionals, and practitioners in the field. We then must rely on those services and institutions for single sensory loss to advocate for us and our complicated access to information, ways of communicating, and support for mobility-orientation. Many in the field of single sensory loss don't understand how DSI means neither sense can compensate for the other. This is hit and miss, and those with DSI are forced to "choose" which is the "primary" disability. Without wider awareness of the distinct disability and its many complexities by structures, researchers, professionals, and practitioners, the wider community remains ignorant and many living with DSI will suffer its impacts in silence. Lack of recognition also promotes data invisibility as well as keeping the personal experiences hidden from view. Finally, in times of austerity and limited budgets, scant data and limited metrics mean that the complex needs of the DSI population are not funded adequately, or simply not funded at all. Such a situation of low recognition fosters marginalization of a rapidly growing group of people globally, nationally, and locally. This is indeed an "invisible epidemic".

Definition

This book is underpinned by the comprehensive Nordic definition of DSI, which identifies DSI as a separate and unique disability:

> Deafblindness is a distinct disability. It is a combined vision and hearing disability. It limits activities of a person and restricts full participation in society to such a degree that society is required to facilitate specific services, environmental alterations and/or technology
>
> (Deafblind Nordic Cooperation Committee, n.d)

The Nordic definition comes with explanatory notes to capture the consequences, complexities, and implications of living with DSI. We reproduce an abridgment of these key complexities of deafblindness–DSI from Watharow (2023) here:

- Distinct and complex disability;
- Hard for each sense to compensate for the other;
- Time consuming;
- Energy draining;
- Activity limiting;
- Participation reducing;
- Information is received in fragments;
- Communication, access to information, and mobility are affected;
- Tactile sense is critical as a conduit of information; and
- Communication technology, assistive devices, interpreters, and adaptations to the environment may be required.

And even acknowledging the above, it is human assistance and supports that remain critical to accessing information, communicating, and promoting mobility and safety.

Most importantly, societal funding to provide all supports needed is essential.

Subtypes of DSI

Age is an accepted defining factor in differentiating DSI population subgroups. There are four developmentally distinct groups acknowledged in the following sections.

Congenital deafness and blindness

Congenital presentations of DSI are those people born with deafness and blindness or combinations of congenital deafness or blindness with a second sensory loss acquired in the prelingual stage (generally birth to two years), which means before the acquisition of speech and language skills. Congenital deafblindness is rare, occurring in 1:29,000 births (Dammeyer, 2010). Causation in this group includes sensory loss/es from intrauterine infections (such as rubella syndrome 28.3 percent) and chromosomal abnormalities (CHARGE syndrome: 20 percent, where CHARGE stands for coloboma, heart defect, atresia choanae, growth retardation, genital, and ear abnormalities). Down syndrome is responsible for 7.9 percent with perinatal asphyxia accounting for 14.3 percent, and prematurity for 7.1 percent (Dammeyer, 2012). While changes in antenatal care and screening are decreasing rates of infections, birth asphyxia, and chromosomal abnormalities, the numbers of babies surviving moderate to extreme prematurity and low to very low birth weights with sensory losses is rising (Hirvonen et al., 2018).

Congenital deafness and acquired vision loss

Around 50 percent of those under 65 years of age with DSI will have congenital deafness with acquired blindness/low vision in the first or second decade of life from retinitis pigmentosa. This combination is known as Usher syndrome and is autosomal recessive. Some subtypes of the syndrome are accompanied by balance disturbances as well as DSI. While there is much research activity, there is presently no cure.

Congenital blindness and acquired hearing loss

This refers to those born with blindness/low vision who acquire hearing loss after a period of hearing. Little data exist on this group but it is rare.

Acquired DSI

This is the most common subgroup. Acquired DSI refers more broadly to the onset of DSI in either early or late life, where language has been developed and the challenge is to maintain communication skills. The majority of people living with acquired DSI are older people. By older people we mean not only those over 65 years of age as per the Australian Institute of Health and Welfare (2019), but also those aging prematurely such as prisoners and the homeless. In addition, First Nations peoples who acquire sensory losses at earlier ages (usually considered over 50 years) are also included in the older age population group when discussing DSI.

Furthermore, Simcock (2017) notes five specifically distinct sub-groups in the older age group with DSI, to this we would add a further category to include hidden populations with premature aging (Simcock: personal communication, 12 December 2023):

a.   Those who have developed DSI in older age (>65 years). This is the aging **into** DSI group and is the largest of the subgroups;

b.   Older people who have vision loss and later develop a hearing loss;

c.   Older people with hearing loss who use speech to communicate, who then develop a vision loss;

d.   Older, culturally deaf people who use sign language, who then develop vision loss;

e.   Older people who have been deafblind for all or most of their life. This is the aging **with** DSI group; and

f.   People with DSI under 65 who are defined as prematurely aging (early or accelerated aging) owing to disadvantageous situations, marginalization, and/or oppression, for example First Nations peoples, those in prison, and homeless people may experience sensory loss/es from the age of 50 (Avery, 2020; Maxmen, 2019). Prisoners, for example, experience premature aging; a 50-year-old person in prison has an equivalent health status (including sensory loss/es) to a 65-year-old in the general population (Trotter and Baidawi, 2015).

This book includes lived experience excerpts from subgroups a–e.

DSI data

To understand how common DSI is in older age, it is important to look at single sensory impairment data. These show the relentless march of sensory loss through life's stages and situate DSI as a growing group in the population, an invisible epidemic, in fact. Separately, vision and hearing loss are identified as significant priorities for the global aging population. Examining the march of single sensory loss in older age demonstrates just how many people are vulnerable to the impact of a second sensory loss.

Hearing loss

The recent *World report on hearing* (WHO, 2021c) identifies hearing loss as the third largest cause of years lived with disability (Global Burden of Disease, 2016; WHO, 2021c). Hearing loss increases with age, impacts communication participation and spatial awareness, and compromises interaction with the environment (Brennan and Bally, 2007; Deafblind Australia, 2016; Scarinci et al., 2008; Schneider et al., 2012; Strawbridge et al., 2000; Wallhagen, 2009; Wallhagen et al., 2008).

Hearing loss affects large numbers of older Australians. Overall hearing loss accounts for 38 percent of all disability types in Australia, reported to the Survey of Disability, Aging and Carers (2019). These data are likely an under representation given that First Nations peoples and remote dwellers are not fully represented. Predictions are that by 2050, one in four will have hearing loss; hearing health is an urgent national priority (House of Representatives Standing Committee on Health, Aged Care and Sport, 2017). The same report found that 66 percent of adults over 60 years had hearing loss, with Dyke (2013) estimating this rising to 75 percent of those over 70 years in Australia.

The pandemic has also highlighted how some, especially older adults with mild hearing loss who previously coped with lipreading and facial cues to augment partially heard information, struggle with the loss of these alongside the muffling of speech by facemasks and shields. This is especially pronounced in hospital, healthcare, and educational settings. Furthermore, the World Health Organization (WHO, 2021c) has warned that one billion young people risk their hearing with damage from high noise levels of earbuds, headphones, and other such devices. There is scant public messaging to warn young users of the risks.

There are many and diverse causes of hearing loss from birth to older age:

- Prenatal period
  - Genetic factors
  - Intrauterine infections
- Perinatal period
  - Birth asphyxia
  - Hyperbilirubinemia
  - Low birth weight
  - Other perinatal morbidities
- Childhood and adolescence
  - Chronic ear infections (chronic suppurative otitis media)
  - Collection of fluid in the ear (chronic non-suppurative otitis media)
  - Meningitis
  - Other infections
- Adulthood and older age
  - Chronic diseases
  - Smoking
  - Otosclerosis
  - Age-related sensorineural degeneration
  - Sudden sensorineural hearing loss

- Factors across the lifespan
  - Trauma to the ear or the head
  - Loud noise/loud sounds
  - Ototoxic medications
  - Work related ototoxic chemicals
  - Nutritional deficiencies
  - Viral infections.

(WHO, 2021a)

Vision loss

Low vision is a global emergency with much of it remediable or reversible (WHO, 2021a). In developing countries up to 50 percent of vision loss is remediable. The 2019 *World report on vision* (WHO, 2019) acknowledges the impact of vision loss in older adults, reporting that blindness is ranked as one of "the most feared ailments, often more so than conditions such as cancer" (p. 15). Vision loss compromises receptive communication, with significant and pervasive impacts on all aspects of everyday life (Brennan and Bally, 2007; Burton et al., 2015; Davis et al., 2016; WHO, 2019).

From the Survey of Disability, Aging and Carers (SDAC, 2019), we know that one percent of Australians live with vision loss that is uncorrectable by wearing glasses. However, 4.6 percent of First Nations people have vision loss and that increases to 13.6 percent of those over 50 years of age (Foreman et al., 2017). Age-related macular degeneration affects 27 percent of all Australians over 80 years of age.

Multiple disability is extremely common: two thirds of Australians with partial or total sight loss report having additional impairments (SDAC, 2019)

Causation of vision loss varies markedly between the Global North and South. Infections and remediable causes predominate in the global south. However, regardless of nationality, age is the strongest predictor of vision loss. Common causes documented by the WHO (2019b) report include:

- Uncorrected refractive errors;
- Cataract/s;
- Age-related macular degeneration;
- Glaucoma;
- Diabetic retinopathy;
- Corneal opacity;
- Strabismus;
- Accident and injury to the eye;
- Tumors (such as retinoblastomas and optic gliomas);
- Vascular occlusions; and
- Retinitis pigmentosa.

(WHO, 2021c)

DSI

The prevalence of DSI is generally hampered by under diagnosis, under reporting, and the invisibility of population groups, such as First Nations peoples, veterans, prisoners, those with multiple disabilities, residents in aged-care facilities, and older Australians who don't recognize their losses as a distinct condition that can be supported and ameliorated. The World Federation for the Deafblind began to collect global data on prevalence to attempt to rectify the knowledge and data gap to produce an estimate of pan-national prevalence. From the 2018 report, we see that

0.2–2 percent of the world's population live with DSI (WFDB, 2018). Most are more than 65 years of age. They are a diverse yet often hidden population, more likely to live in poverty, experience under employment, and be less educated (WFDB, 2018).

In China, using self-reporting of DSI, Heine, Gong and Browning, (2019) found that 57.2 percent of older adults (>60 years) experienced DSI in a cross-sectional analysis of data from the China Health and Retirement Longitudinal Study.

In Australia, data from Senses Australia in 2013 put the number of Australians living with DSI at 100,000 (5:100). Yet, from the SDAC (2019), even though there is no recognition of DSI as a distinct and unique disability, as well as poor inclusion of First Nations peoples and those living in remote regions, 200,000 people of all age groups are estimated to have a combined full or partial hearing loss with a full or partial vision loss. This equates to a rate of 8:1000 Australians in 2019 living with DSI. Schneider et al. (2012) noted that the prevalence of DSI increased significantly with very old age to 26.8 percent in those aged >80 years. This confirms the data shift of increasing rates of DSI as the population ages (Mick et al., 2021; Schneider et al., 2012). Data from the Canadian Longitudinal Study on Aging (which does not include prisoners or targeted indigenous inclusion), noted that the prevalence of DSI increased from 8.7 percent in 2011 to 16.9 percent in 2016, due to population aging and growth (Mick et al., 2021).

Worryingly, the trend observed by Heine and Browning in 2002 that existing services and structures did not meet the needs of people, carers, and families living with DSI continues two decades on (Dunsmore, 2022).

Causation

Acquired DSI in older age (or a decade earlier if in susceptible subpopulations as mentioned previously) is increasing sharply, in line with population aging (Mick et al., 2021; Tiwana et al., 2016). The key causes of DSI in those over 65 years are commonly age-related conditions such as age-related macular degeneration, cataract, glaucoma, and presbycusis (age- related loss) (Guthrie et al., 2016; Heine and Browning, 2015; Schneider et al., 2011). But, as seen from the causation lists of single sensory loses earlier, any condition that causes hearing loss and any condition that results in low vision means a person acquiring DSI.

Severity

There is wide heterogeneity in the severity of DSI, with combinations ranging from mild to complete sensory loss in either or both senses. There is a Deafblindness Severity Index (Dalby et al., 2009) but this is not in wide use in the older age population.

To date, inconsistent measurement of DSI and a lack of a common international definition compromises research translation between professionals in health, education, and research (Larsen and Damen, 2014; Schneider et al., 2011; Wittich et al., 2013). In a systematic review of DSI in older adults, Heine and Browning (2015) reported methods to measure DSI which ranged from objective measurements (such as the Snellen letter test chart, visual field examination, pure tone audiometry) to self-report measures (response to questions). Further complicating any assessment of "severity" are the impacts of co-morbidities and other impairments, variable individual and family resources, diversity in personal coping, and that nations have different recognition of and support for those living with DSI. There is presently work underway by the WHO on their International Classification of Functioning (ICF) to document the specific complexities of deafblindness–DSI (Wittich, W. (Personal Communication, July, 2023)).

An aging population means a growing population living with DSI: An invisible epidemic

The global aging population is the fastest growing age demographic, with predictions that by 2050 those aged over 60 years will represent 22 percent of the total global population; likewise, those aged >80 years are expected to triple by 2050, reaching 426 million (WHO, 2021a). A baby born today is predicted to live until 100 years of age. In line with global projections, the proportion of the Australian population aged >65 years increased from 12.4 percent in 2000 to 16.3 percent in 2020; in the same period, the number of older adults >85 years increased by 110 percent (Australian Bureau of Statistics [ABS], 2020). Population aging is testament to medical advances and social improvements in the last 50 years; however, there are costs to "living longer" as noted by the concomitant increases in chronic non-communicable diseases (e.g., type 2 diabetes, obesity, and osteoarthritis) and rates of disabilities such as DSI (Beard et al., 2016; Maresova et al., 2019; WHO, 2015). These demographic changes shape global health needs, with an increasing focus on prevention and social determinants of health, and a renewed focus on healthier aging and optimizing function in older people (WHO, 2020).

Additionally, both WHO world reports on hearing and vision draw immediate attention to the greater burden of disability experienced in low- to middle-income nations and indigenous global populations. This is consistent with recent studies in two populous nations, India (Jaiswal et al., 2020; Marmamula et al., 2021) and Malaysia (Mah et al., 2020).

Based on current population aging trajectories, the prevalence of DSI is projected to increase significantly. Additionally, and, because females tend to live longer than males, a greater burden may be experienced by women, particularly those aged >80 years (AIHW, 2020; Heine et al., 2019).

Invisible populations

Hidden from the view of data collectors and researchers are sub-populations of those with single sensory loss or DSI. This renders current data as underestimates. These invisible older populations include but are not limited to: older people with unrecognized/unacknowledged DSI; residents in aged-care facilities; veterans; prisoners; First Nations peoples; the homeless; and those living with other or multiple disabilities.

Unrecognized/unacknowledged DSI

Older people may not self-report as having DSI. As mentioned earlier they may regard sensory loss as an inevitable part of aging. Professionals busy with the complex needs of older patients may not check hearing and vision parameters among other chronic conditions and impairments. Older adults may experience stigma and fail to disclose sensory loss and its associated difficulties (Dunsmore, 2022). In addition, given the need for care for persons with DSI, it is important to note that family carers often do not understand or recognize the complexities of DSI, tending to minimize impacts, or normalize as simply "part of aging."This has serious implications for interpersonal relationships and maintaining social engagement. This is explored in detail in Chapters 5 and 6.

Residents of aged-care facilities

Guthrie et al., (2022) notes that among older adults in long term care, DSI is the most common sensory loss outstripping single sensory loss. Yet, an alarming number of residents live with undiagnosed sensory loss/es (Pavey et al., 2009). This Sense UK commissioned study of eight residential aged-care facilities found that approximately 30 percent of those living in residential aged-care facilities had undiagnosed DSI.

Other and multiple disabilities are common and increase with advancing age. The WFDB (2018) estimates that 25–75 percent of people with DSI have other disability/ies and this increases with age. In Residential Aged Care Facilities (RACF), multiple disability is the norm, and so DSI may be undetected.

Veterans

Data are held on only a small percentage of Australian ex-defense forces personnel, so much remains unknown. However, sensory losses are common concomitants of military service due to injury and noise exposure. Hussain et al. (2021) reported that 38 percent of a military population with traumatic brain injuries from their service had moderate to severe vision loss. Exposure to military noise such as blast trauma leads to high rates of occupational hearing loss in serving military personnel and veterans (Australian Government, 2017). Under recognition of sensory losses is common in American military populations (Smith, Bennett and Wilson, 2008).

Prisoners

It is well documented that prisoners experience accelerated aging and sensory losses. As a group they are predominately older, male, with First Nations peoples overrepresented. Trotter and Badawi (2015), estimated that a 50-year-old male prisoner had the health status of a 65-year-old in the general population.

First Nations peoples

A historically neglected group, First Nations peoples live with high rates of sensory loss, and these losses develop earlier in age. Avery (2020) for example, reported 82 percent of First Nations people over 50 years have hearing loss of which 66 percent is unreported: meaning that hearing loss develops earlier but is not identified or supported. Foreman et al. (2017), noted that First Nations peoples develop vision loss up to 15 years earlier and at twice or more the rate of other Australians. Dyke (2013) suggested that 42 percent of First Nations people live with single or dual sensory loss. Both Dyke (2013) and the Australian Government, House of Representatives Report (2017) noted that much of this sensory loss is preventable. Issues with access to health diagnosis and care, intersectionality, double disadvantage, racism, and diagnostic overshadowing mean invisibility in the current data. See Avery, Culture is Inclusion (2018) for more on disability, data, and the complexities experienced by First Nations people.

Homeless

This is a population that experiences an accelerated aging process (that includes sensory loss/es) alongside poor data and support services (Maxmen, 2019). There are no data on DSI in this group that we could find.

Multiple disability

Sensory loss/es may be invisible in the presence of other impairments such as dementia, traumatic brain injuries (Hussain et al., 2021), and intellectual disability (Fellinger et al., 2009). Diagnostic overshadowing may occur where the impacts of undiagnosed sensory loss are blamed on other disabilities (Blair, 2019). Single and DSI should be regularly considered in older adults especially in the presence of other conditions.

Conclusion

We have shown here the relentless march of sensory losses in older age. Yet while DSI is increasingly common, policy, practices, and available supports are inadequate for the task of supporting individuals, carers, and families. DSI is a distinct disability and confers many complexities and difficulties for those living with the condition, as well as those caring for and/or living with them. The next chapter will look at some of the impacts on health, well-being, and security (Chapter 3). Throughout this book we challenge the idea that DSI is something to be tolerated in silence or shame.

3

Dual sensory impairment

Health, well-being, and security

Introduction

The invisible epidemic of dual sensory impairment (DSI) in older adults poses a significant threat to health, well-being, and security, particularly if we are not adequately supported. We will look now at some of the challenges for older people, both aging *with* and aging *into* DSI. These are not exhaustive but indicative of the complicated potential flow on effects of living with DSI in older age, especially if poorly supported and resourced. It shouldn't be this way, and it doesn't have to be. In Chapter 11 we will examine the experiences of an older adult with DSI which will provide some pragmatic recommendations beyond the research.

A note on vulnerability

We advise readers that while this chapter discusses threats, risks, and vulnerabilities, we do not mean to imply that living with DSI means being in a constant negative state of vulnerability. We see vulnerability as situational and therefore, dynamic. People may enter, exit, and re-enter situations where they experience risk to health or well-being. Being hospitalized is one example of a situational vulnerability but it is not the sensory losses that comprise the threat, it is the failure of care and communication by health professionals and institutions that increase the likelihood of risk.

All these extensive risks may sound alarming and precarious, but the provision of good social and human supports means that older people with DSI have the capacity to live better and longer.

Health, well-being, and security

DSI can impact communication, access to healthcare and personal experiences of that care; physical health; public health; psychological well-being; and cognitive health. DSI also poses a risk to our sense of safety and security of the self; and this ontological insecurity contributes to difficulties navigating life with DSI as an older person. There is a major gap in our understanding of the impact on the health, well-being, and security of families and carers.

Communication

Good communication lets people with DSI know what is happening, and confers a positive sense of health benefits, fostering the advancement of health, security, and safety. Communication disruption as a consequence of sensory losses means that neither sense is able to compensate for the other, leading to increased stress during social situations, increasing dependence on others to navigate social and physical environments, and a reluctance to engage socially (Erber and Scherer, 1999; Heine and Browning, 2002, 2004).

Family carers often provide this day-to-day support to aid communication, navigate public spaces, including the healthcare system, and manage activities of daily living. There is significant and often unrecognized effort in this carer support, and often the social effort, the concern for safety, and interpersonal tension limits opportunities for social engagements for both. Multiple missed social opportunities create resentment and exacerbate interpersonal tension, often due to a mismatch of expectations between needs of caregiver and care receiver. Much of this is related to misunderstanding of DSI and the perception that those with DSI could "try harder" as they are not "fully blind and deaf" (family carers' narratives, Dunsmore, 2022). This lack of understanding is pervasive more broadly and consideration should be directed to understanding the complex, multifactorial consequences that impact both family carer and person with DSI.

Health and poor communication

Poor communication also decreases patient safety and is linked to negative outcomes. See Slade et al. (2015) for a substantial, real-world examination of these in hospital emergency departments, and Eggins et al. (2016) for the pitfalls of poor communication in handovers in clinical settings. Both show how effective communication improves patient safety, care, and access to information. However, accommodations and accessibility provisions can only occur when sensory losses are known. It has been established that sensory impairment information is poorly documented in medical records (Dullard and Saunders, 2016), but, even if well documented, staff often fail to read these notes (Watharow, 2021).

A report by Sense UK 2016 found deafblind people were failed by health services, with half not understanding the procedures they had. In Australia, 89 percent of participants with DSI did not understand what professionals and service providers in hospital told them (Watharow, 2023). These findings devalue person-centered care, shared decision making, and informed consent. Indeed, no participant in Watharow's (2021) study received a consent form considered accessible to them. Participants like Tom said they signed their consent form "not knowing what was on it".

Poor communication for any patient is linked to:

- More frequent hospital stays;
- Longer length of stays;
- More frequent readmissions to hospital;
- More visits to emergency departments;
- Poor adherence and understanding of treatment;
- Less frequent medical follow up; and
- Poorer health and well-being outcomes generally (Slade et al., 2015).

And because of the way institutions and professionals fail to provide access to information, person-centered care, and communication support, hospitals place patients with DSI at greater risk and actuality of harm (Watharow, 2021). Hersh (2013) too, reminds us that it is not the impairments themselves posing the risk but rather the lack of accommodation and understanding by attendants.

These failures impact healthcare costs so there is a cost benefit to institutions and professionals to reduce economic burden by improving communication and care. Research by Huddle et al. (2016) has quantified both single and dual sensory impairment in the USA, as a significant increase to cost and healthcare burden. They note that attention to sensory impairments with diagnosis, support, and remediation would see major health cost reductions. In addition, communication lies at the heart of most adverse medical events, and are expensive (Slade et al., 2015). Patients with sensory loss are among the most exposed to these communication misadventures (Bartlett et al., 2008).

Communication and assistive devices

Hearing aids are a polarizing assistive device for communication. On one hand, hearing aids that are well fitted and well received confer benefits of improved communication, social participation, and longer life. Choi et al. (2024) found that people regularly wearing hearing aids regardless of degree of loss, age, gender, insurance status, and presence of other medical conditions, lived longer (24% lower mortality risk than people with hearing loss who never wore hearing aids). There is also ongoing research suggesting that wearing hearing aids may mitigate the risk for those with hearing loss of cognitive decline (Bucholc et al., 2021; Jiang et al., 2023) The mechanisms are poorly understood or defined but worth considering.

Hearing aid use is not as widely practiced as the wearing of glasses and is often stigmatized. There are very recent reports in the popular press, for example, Bloomberg Business Week, December 6, 2023, of changes that may increase user acceptability where ear bud companies are investing in creating hearing amplification versions. As ear buds are considered widely acceptable, particularly with younger demographics, the outlet predicts that "Hearing aids are about to be as common as reading glasses".

Complicating factors in hearing aid use include:

- Misconceptions: These abound around hearing loss, aids, cochlear implants, and communication among professionals, practitioners, family members, and carers, and more broadly, in society. It is often suggested that the impairment is "solved" or "cured" with hearing aids, and that adaptations, adjustments, rehabilitation and assistance are no longer required. Other misconceptions may include: i) "everyone can have a cochlear implant"; ii) "cochlear implants mean normal hearing"; iii) "hearing aids mean normal hearing"; iv) "hearing aids always work in every setting".

- Hearing assistive technologies have many challenges in practice, for example, batteries may run out, moulds may get blocked, air around loose moulds or fractured tubing may create interference. Some unwanted sounds are amplified, and some wanted sounds are muted which can result in communication tensions, failures, and misunderstandings. Author A has hearing aids and can hear the rustling of their hair over the aid but not the sound of voices on the phone. A common complaint among older people is that hearing devices in fact make hearing conversations in parties and gatherings worse.

- Barriers to continued wearing of aids from lived experience of older people with sensory losses, include:

  "The tiny knobs too small for old fingers... and so difficult to get the sticky paper off the back of the batteries"
  "My hearing aid whistles"

"My hearing aid keeps falling out"

"I dropped my hearing aid into water and now it doesn't work"

"My hearing aid keeps buzzing"

"I can't remember the different programs…it's too complicated"

"My friends make fun of me"

"I can't find my hearing aids because I can't see".

These barriers mean that hearing rehabilitation needs to be person centered, flexible, and ongoing (Boisvert et al., 2022).

Communication and Covid-19

The Covid-19 pandemic has had a further negative effect on communication for many. Ubiquitous mask wearing, often in combination with face shields has muffled sounds and eliminated facial cues and lipreading. This means that those who managed communication encounters with residual senses (by using lipreading and facial cues) became more impaired.

Loss of communication partners and social networks

People living with DSI are at risk of social isolation as a consequence of ineffective communication and loss of social networks. Social isolation compromises health and well-being in insidious ways (see Dunsmore, (2022) for a fuller exploration of this and also Chapter 5). Research links social isolation to greater rates of depression, low sleep quality, impaired executive functioning, cognitive decline, poor cardiovascular function, and impaired immunity at every stage in life (Hawkley and Capitanio, 2015). So, attention and investment in communication is urgently needed to stem the tide of social isolation for the increasing numbers of those living with DSI.

Access to healthcare

People with disability generally experience reduced access to health services which impacts their health and well-being (Berghs et al., 2016). People with DSI experience less access than both sighted-hearing people and those with other disabilities (WFDB, 2018). Older people with DSI experience difficulties navigating social welfare systems, accessing healthcare, and managing their own health risks. There are significant barriers to participation for those with DSI, which are pervasive and intersectional. Ageism, stigma, and personal concerns about increasing dependency limit participation; barriers to participation extend to reduced access to large organizations such as healthcare systems, and the need for accompaniment to appointments (Mick et al., 2018; Reed et al., 2020). The need for assistance during healthcare interactions is generally addressed by family (or informal) carers who provide the majority of health and social care for those with DSI in Australia (ABS, 2018; Dyke, 2013; Kelley et al., 2017) (For further exploration of the role of family carers, see Chapters 5 and 6). In addition to these difficulties with access to services, poor experiences often equate to delayed health help-seeking behaviors; as one participant said, "I will never go back there [to hospital] no matter what" (Watharow, 2021).

Few dedicated health and social care services for DSI

Fragmentation of health services further complicates access to information and care (Schneider et al., 2012). The absence of recognition of DSI as a unique and distinct disability means that there may be a single impairment focus and these services may have poor understandings and/or limited resources available for the complex needs of DSI. What this means is that there are few support services that specialize in DSI. Consequently, people with DSI do not have access to best practice support for their combined sensory loss. Takahashi's (2019) presentation noted the lack of professional understanding of deafblindness as a key concern for Japanese people living with DSI.

The difficulty accessing appropriate health services for people living with DSI exacerbates the risk of mental health issues (Bodsworth, Clare and Simblett, 2011). These difficulties result in unmet needs and "sadness, helplessness, anxiety, depression and withdrawal" (Bodsworth et al., 2011, p. 7). DSI and psychological well-being will be discussed later in the chapter.

Experiences of healthcare

People with DSI are more likely to need healthcare support and hospitalization than those without (Hajek and König, 2020; Huddle et al., 2016), but are more likely to experience reduced access and negative experiences during their healthcare encounters with negative touch, neglect, dehumanization, and restrictive practices reported (Takahashi, 2019; Watharow, 2023).

Good communication is the most significant factor in positive patient experiences (Cunnett, 2010) and good experiences are strongly linked to improved health and well-being (Sutherland et al., 2017). Notwithstanding the moral and ethical imperatives, better communication and positive health experiences save money. Accordingly, efforts to improve communication and relational aspects of care need to be seen as a good investment.

Physical health threats

Studies show DSI compromises health-related quality of life (Kwon et al., 2015; Tseng et al., 2018) but there is limited knowledge on exactly how and why. Threats to health may come from the environment, the conditions causing DSI, the functional decline associated with DSI, and even the DSI itself.

Threats from the environment

There are many threats from the environment as sensory loss leads to lower awareness of environmental warning signals such as hearing traffic noise and sirens, seeing obstacles, stairs, and escalators. There is a higher risk of traffic accidents as both pedestrians and drivers. Accidents are more common in homes, for example, with hot water, tea, and coffee leading to scalds and burns. In Watharow (2021), falls and accidents were responsible for the hospital admission of one third of study participants.

Reduced food and medication safety

Low vision can lead to poor food safety resulting in gastrointestinal illness. Low vision can lead to misreading medication labels. Poor communication by health professionals can result in misunderstanding health instructions and this poses a risk to physical health and well-being. As Robert says "three, thirteen, thirty, or thirty-three all sound the same. And the more the better right?" Not true for medication: if you are on three units of insulin, thirty-three may prove fatal.

Risks from conditions causing DSI and treatment

These include: Usher syndrome, which has high rates of cataracts.

Cochlear implantation is an invasive procedure with a small risk of adverse events (Gheorghe and Zamfir-Chru-Anton, 2015). These are more the province of those aging with DSI.

Multiple disability and chronic age-related health conditions pose additional risks for those living and aging with DSI. These additional impairments add complexity to functional capacity, as well as health and well-being.

DSI and functional decline

Individuals with DSI are at increased risk of functional decline due to the loss of the compensatory mechanism of one sense over another (Davidson and Guthrie, 2019). This interrupts inter-action with the physical and social environment and compro-mises the capacity of older persons to complete activities of daily living including more complex instrumental activities (Brennan and Bally, 2007; Brennan et al., 2005; Guthrie et al., 2018; Heine and Browning, 2015). In a recent study from Korea, community dwelling older people with DSI had lower muscle mass, with decreased physical health and functioning, compared to their non-impaired counterparts (Kong et al., 2023). This suggests that DSI may stimulate a complex cascade of events that impact physi-cal health and well-being for older adults. Currently, there are few DSI-specific validated tools for assessing older people: only one tool validated for patients with DSI currently exists for functional impairment with a deafblind supplement (Alfaro et al., 2021).

Public health threats

Good public health awareness is founded on good communication. Those with communication or cultural differences are adversely impacted if not purposefully accommodated and included. Not seeing or hearing public health messages can be a risk to health: for example, not being aware of influenza vaccination means missing out on potential protection against serious illness. This was particularly well highlighted during the recent Covid-19 pandemic with problematic messaging and health management for many with disabilities, including those with DSI (Shakespeare, 2021).

Public health research is also less inclusive of people with disability generally, and particularly those with sensory losses (Berghs et al., 2016). The key drivers of this exclusion include failure to obtain lived experience testimonies and a reliance instead on professional observations, assessments, and proxy reports. Older adults often have a different self-assessment of their risks, priorities, and safety from the professionals involved in their care (Abley et al., 2011). The failure to provide accessible formats for research in public health and other domains, as well as ableist methodologies, excludes those who need adjustments and accommodations (Watharow and Wayland, 2022). This results in testimonial injustices and contributes to ongoing data invisibility of affected populations. Data invisibility means poorly conceived and allocated supports to those who are in most need. This issue of invisibility impacts protection, policies, professional education, and practices not only in public health, but more widely in social care and healthcare.

Poor inclusion in disaster preparation and response

Inadequate government responses, services, and disaster management compromise the health and well-being of those with disability, those who are older, and those with DSI (Leach and Scully, 2020; Shakespeare, 2021). Racism, ableism, and ageism have marred the disaster discourse and response, and the Covid-19 virus was particularly lethal to older people, and those in residential aged-care facilities.

Some of the public discussion centered around the expendability of older people and rationing of health resources away from people with disability and/or older citizens (Andrews et al., 2021). It was particularly evident in Australia that the prolonged lack of investment in aged-care infrastructure impacted many older persons in residential aged care. Fukuyama (2020) highlights that robust social care institutions were a key factor in countries with a good pandemic response. For people living in residential aged care, the pandemic has been a disaster fueled by ageism, ableism, and racism which in part contributed to high mortality and morbidity in at risk groups, especially older citizens and those living with disability.

There has been research that indicates that recent natural disasters and the Covid pandemic planning and responses have not been informed by people with disability, and older people with DSI specifically (Villeneuve et al., 2021). This neglect, in combination with testimonial injustices and data invisibility has compromised the health and well-being of people affected by disasters (Villeneuve et al., 2021).

For a better approach to inclusive disaster preparations and response see Villeneuve et al. (2021) regarding applying a person-centered capability framework to inform targeted action on disability inclusive disaster risk reduction.

Exclusion

New ways of living, accelerated by the pandemic such as online shopping, entertainment, and digital healthcare have not been universally beneficial to older people with DSI. Those with DSI may lack the resources, devices, connectivity, dexterity, and familiarity with online platforms. Some do not have enough residual hearing and sight to navigate the digital world. This means they are exiled from the new mainstream modes of communicating, with reduced access to telehealth services and online social support. This directly compromises the health, well-being, and security of older people with DSI.

Psychological well-being

There is a wealth of literature that establishes a relationship between DSI and reduced psychological and cognitive well-being. Bodsworth et al. (2011) note high rates of psychological distress among those with DSI across all age groups. Research centered on older adults has consistently demonstrated that the consequences of DSI extend beyond daily function and communication, with strong links to depression (Capella-McDonnall, 2005; Heine and Browning, 2015; Heine et al., 2019; Lupsakko et al., 2002). Moderate rates of depression and anxiety are seen in 60- to 90-year-olds with DSI (Figueiredo, Chiari and Goulart, 2013). Ontological insecurity likely plays a role in psychological distress and will be explored shortly.

There are complex pathways between DSI and psychological well-being, and these are not well understood. Is there a biological factor the predisposes people with DSI, or is it that having DSI on its own compromises psychological functioning? And what about social isolation? What role does this play in well-being?

Some of the tools used in evaluating and diagnosing psychological or cognitive conditions may not be validated for patients with sensory impairments. This may result in incorrect diagnoses and treatments (Shen et al., 2020).

Cognitive health

There is much recent literature on the risk of single and dual sensory impairments increasing the risk of cognitive decline (Davidson and Guthrie, 2019; Schneider et al., 2011; Lin et al., 2004; Livingston et al., 2020; Mukadam 2018; Jaiswal et al., 2020). Jiang et al. (2023) have suggested that hearing aid wearing reduces the risk of cognitive decline to normal, non-impaired levels. There is also a suggestion by Bucholc et al. (2021) and others, that hearing aids decrease dementia risks. While the mechanisms are poorly understood, the association with cognitive decline appears strong resulting in growing global concern.

On the other hand, the presence of sensory loss/es can lead to the incorrect diagnoses of cognitive decline. People with sensory loss may appear to have a cognitive impairment when, for example, they do not hear the questions being asked of them and score poorly on mental state examinations. This may have a chain of consequence with incorrect treatments and tests (Shen et al., 2020). Robert, for example, is diagnosed with dementia when a mini mental state examination is performed when he doesn't have his hearing aids in, or accommodations for his low vision made.

Delirium

Delirium is common in those with single and DSI (Ahmed et al., 2014). This is a condition where an alteration in attention, awareness, perception, and cognition is experienced. Delirium commonly complicates care in the acute setting of hospitalization after falls, fractures, and infections.

Visual hallucinations

Visual hallucinations are very common and around one third of those with low vision may experience these. However, awareness and supports are low resulting in few being diagnosed and reassured as to the benign nature of their experiences. This is known as Charles Bonnet syndrome and will be detailed in the following chapter. Visual hallucinations are distressing and commonly misattributed to cognitive conditions.

Tinnitus

Tinnitus is an "invisible" but commonly occurring symptom that refers to the perception of sound in the absence of any external stimulus. This is often described as a ringing or buzzing in the ears. A fuller examination of tinnitus and its consequences will follow in Chapter 4).

Ontological security and well-being

The concept of ontological security as used here derives from the work of R.D Laing (1965) and Giddens (1991). Ontological security is the fundamental sense of safety, reliability, and trust in people, places, and things. Laing asserts that a sense of security is necessary to navigate the "hazards of life" (Laing, 1965, p. 39). Communication and access to trustworthy information and people is critical for ontological security development and maintenance. The consequences of loss of this security and trust are "Greater anxieties and dangers" (Laing, 1965, p. 67) and "chaos…. and a loading in of anxiety" (Giddens, 1991, p. 36). Laing and Giddens establish a clear link between ontologically insecure states and psychological health harms. Navigating life's hazards as Laing describes it, or problem solving and decision making, requires the security of trustworthy information and people. These can be compromised for people living with DSI as the very nature of the condition centers around fragmented information, fraught communication, and disorienting environments.

Hersh (2013) notes that for people with DSI, informed decision making requires clear information, good communication, and an appropriate environment for the delivery of that information. For older people with DSI, the combined impairments of sight and hearing mean that we cannot always trust what we see and hear which leads to feeling "vulnerable, insecure and unconfident" (Heine and Browning, 2004, p. 116), particularly in older age.

We will briefly examine the experiences of older people with DSI to highlight the ontological insecurity experienced. These include unpredictable people, trust, privacy, and information. "Not knowing what is going on" is one state of ontological insecurity.

Unpredictable people

We have alluded previously to the difficulties for people with DSI in their engagement with healthcare professionals, (such as doctors and nurses), who may have little experience of communication and accessibility requirements in a DSI context. These present not only threats to safety but risks to psychological well-being.

Dunsmore writes extensively about how the loss of carer/spouse/ families threatens ontological security (2022). Diminishing social networks have a significant impact on health and security; however, the loss of a spouse or close family member who has carer responsibilities, may act as a catalyst to changing circumstances and further social disruption. Losing a spouse often prompted participants to consider decisions about future living arrangements, creating tension for participants as they balanced, for example, the loss of their community against the potential benefits of moving closer to family. This loss poses a threat to security and often signposts a transition between independence and dependence. Viv described the discussions she had with her general practitioner (GP) in England about migration following the death of her husband: "The GP said 'You've lost [husband] and now you're going to lose all your friends. Think about this very carefully'. And I did. And I struggled with that" (Viv) (Dunsmore, 2022, p. 98).

Unpredictable trust

Dunsmore (2022) additionally highlights how situations with new support workers or frequent changes of these, threatens people with DSI and their trust in others. This is particularly seen with external (paid, formal) carers. Trust was integral to success in engaging services and minor incidents could dissuade those with DSI from their ongoing use. Disengagement from services would occur despite the consequences for both participants *and* their families, who were often left filling the gap if services were discontinued. Tony described one such incident where he felt his trust had been abused saying:

> The next time she [worker] came, she just took one [bottle of water] and I said to myself that's not on. If she wanted one, I would have gladly given it to her. Just ask (Tony).
>
> (Dunsmore, 2022, p. 101)

Unpredictable privacy

There are threats to privacy as access to clear information on services was often difficult for participants with DSI, because of complex and visually challenging websites and participants having no clear idea of their own entitlements: Bridget said, "I didn't know where to start with it". This meant that, for some, there was a need to balance the perceived threat to privacy against their pressing need for support.

This lack of predictability has to be balanced against the potential benefits of integrating and building relationships with formal care networks to improve (in this case) the study participants' quality of life. Trustworthy care relationships facilitate access to other external social activities and networks. For more on this please see Chapters 5 and 6.

Unpredictable things

 With vision loss the placement and nature of objects can become less certain and can be deceptive, e.g., blurring with cataracts or loss of depth perception following a vascular event in one eye. This can precipitate accidents and falls and invoke fear and distress.

Unpredictable places

 For those living with DSI it is not only external environments that pose unseen hazards but one's own home can feel unpredictable. This may catalyze the need for additional care and potential early entry to a residential aged-care facility, retirement home, or downsizing. Hospitalizations may present challenges to security and safety as there may be many unfamiliar environments due to frequent bed/ward changes, as well as the multiple hazards of obstacles. William, a participant in Watharow (2021) notes that there are "trolleys and whatnot everywhere on the way to the bathroom".

Residential aged care and risk

Residential aged care is purportedly a place of care and safeguarding. However, the recent Royal Commission into Aged Care Quality and Safety has repeatedly heard, those "homes" are very often places of jeopardy (2021). Older people living with disability are subject to increased rates of violence, abuse, neglect, and exploitation (Commonwealth of Australia, 2021). For further information on this, refer to reports on the Royal Commission into Aged Care Quality and Safety and the Royal Commission into Violence, Abuse, Neglect and Exploitation of People with Disability (Commonwealth of Australia, 2021).

Families and carers

Third party disability, and health and well-being impacts on families and carers remain a major gap in the body of knowledge on DSI. There are limited data on dyadic (family/carer and person with DSI) experiences of access and communication in healthcare (Dunsmore et al., 2020; Kiely et al., 2020).

Conclusion

This book draws attention to the broad lack of visibility of DSI at all levels of society and the risks this poses to health, well-being, and security. The lived experience of DSI is complex and contingent with no recognition as a distinct disability in Australia, unlike both the UK and the EU. This leads to individuals and families like our own, becoming reliant on professionals who may have limited awareness and few targeted resources to provide structured and practical assistance. DSI confers multiple risks to physical, psychological, cognitive, security of the self, and social well-being; we see communication at the heart of this complexity.

Whose responsibility is it to ensure that older people with DSI are supported and safer; that they are as well as possible in body and mind; that they experience effective and accessible communication in all situations; and are provided with true person-centered care in the healthcare system? This responsibility belongs to all of us: to society at large, its institutions, and social support systems. It is the responsibility of healthcare professionals and practitioners to increase their awareness and proficiency in the communication and care of all people with disability, older people in particular. There is a responsibility on lawmakers and policy writers to recognize the distinct disability status of DSI and provide for the complex support needs of those living with DSI, and their families/carers. And wherever possible we need to help ourselves as well by being prepared, by learning new ways of doing and being, and by telling others about our experiences in order that we all learn what works well and what doesn't.

4
Seeing the unseen: Hearing the unheard

Charles Bonnet syndrome and tinnitus

We list the things we don't see that are real:

> Curbs;
> Stairs;
> Suitcases;
> Jetties we fall off. Down. Over. Into; and
> I see things that aren't there, I tell Loretta.

"Me too, me too, she says. There's a small girl in a red coat who appears out of nowhere occasionally. Takes me a while to realize she isn't real. The child wears a coat with a hood and black buttons that pop in the sea of red. I'm always startled but then I look at the little wee thing and say, 'Where is your mummy or daddy?' Then I see her face and it's all distorted, like in a horror movie. Oh, my heart pounds so fast. Why is her face so distorted? After a few minutes I realize she isn't a real child, she isn't a real anything."

I tell Loretta that we, who are losing our sight, are always running into people, places, and things. We're also losing our hearing, so we don't catch the warnings yelled out by family, friends, and passers-by, "Watch out for the lady with the stroller, the man with the dog, the rubbish bin, the edge of the jetty, the ornamental pond, the toys on the carpet, the crawling baby almost underfoot…".

Loretta says, "Exactly, and this means whenever I 'see' the child in the red coat, I react as if she is real until I realize, aha, she is not. I can never tell when she will turn up, or where. She's been in some pretty weird places, like the Bowling Club, the pub toilets, the shed outside the house. She is so clear to me, but, oh my goodness, her face is always just so gruesome as if black paint has leaked onto a watercolor painting and run".

Loretta mentions her visual apparitions started after her sight loss suddenly worsened; about two years ago.

"I ask, does your apparition move, or just stand there.

She answers, that's pretty interesting to think about. I think she just stands there; it is me that is usually moving, walking toward her. It's my startle that makes it seem like she moves. But it is me".

"I know" I say to Loretta, "I've a couple of different hallucinations and they both have moving parts. There's a man in the dark suit with a burgundy tie who has been jack-knifing out at me since I began losing my sight a few decades ago, and the more recent hallucination of an analog watch face that tells a different, but fictitious time whenever I look at it. I have to resort to checking the time on my mobile phone or asking someone what the (real) time is. The man in the dark suit jumps out at me mostly in places with dim lighting: I never see him inside the house when the lights are on, for example. But I do see him in poorly lit streets. He looks like a dark doorway".

"The thing is, he is scary because I think, as women, it is ingrained in us to be careful in dark places and that strange men are regarded as potential threats. So, I'm always frightened. Even if it is transient, whenever I encounter that man. My friend says she can tell when I see him because I jerk suddenly and grasp her arm tightly, sometimes muttering, 'sorry, sorry, sorry', as if I have bumped into someone. His face is pixelated and indistinct, and he himself is not scary (unlike Loretta's phantom child's face). His dark suit has brass buttons that sparkle, the tie is the color of a glass of good red!"

We both keep our visions secret for a long time, our deeply private delusions, surely evidence of imminent dementia or psychotic illness? Neither desirable nor good, especially at our age. Vision loss has upended our lives: Loretta with a vascular eye condition and Meniere's disease, causing hearing loss, and me with lifelong deafness, an inherited eye condition, and a retinal detachment that is unrelated to everything else, but devastating in its impact.

We find that we miss similar things and that the vision loss is "the worst thing ever". We agree that we could manage the hearing loss if that was all we had to contend with. But it is not. Here's some of what we miss:

- Faces, mainly for both of us;
- And books;
- Going out by ourselves is next;

- Having parties for Loretta;
- Traveling and enjoying the local scenery for me; and
- Loretta doesn't miss cooking, but I do, immensely.

On top of these losses, we worry about the things that we see that aren't real.

Loretta says, "my ophthalmologist says 'I have to learn to live with my low vision'. He is so busy, and I'm in and out of there before I can ask him about these 'visions' I'm having. I know enough to know it is not normal and cannot be good but I don't understand exactly what's happening. I eat lots of carrots because they are supposed to be good for eye health. I get new glasses. Nothing makes a difference. The lost child in her red coat still comes. I'm beginning to worry that I will trip when I try to avoid running into her. And all this is on top of worrying, am I going insane?"

I tell Loretta that exactly, yes that is the riptide running under the apparitions. "I *know* I am sane. Really. But still the worry makes me jumpy, forgetful. The Greek chorus in my brain, like Loretta's is chanting dementia, dementia, dementia. Then mad, mad, mad".

When Loretta finally tells her daughter Helen, she mentions, "I know Helen is thinking dementia, dementia, dementia too". Helen books an urgent doctor's appointment, even though I tell her I have been having these "experiences" for a couple of years now. She thinks we need to know why, so that we can "plan and prepare". The GP agrees with my daughter and so begins the carousel of tests, scans and referrals. I'm asked to remember three objects and to count backward by sevens so many times that I practice these when I'm not being tested! There is a bit of a kerfuffle when I mishear the three objects (score zero) because

I forgot my hearing aids, but I get back to 100 percent accuracy with them in. Finally, I reach the psychogeriatrician (who if I understand rightly is a psychiatrist for old folk). I tell her about the coat, the hood, the black buttons, and the grotesque face.

The psychogeriatrician tells me, "Firstly, this is something that is often experienced by people losing their sight, especially older people. It's got a fancy name, Charles Bonnet syndrome. Nothing to worry about".

> So…no dementia then? asks my daughter.
> NO DEMENTIA says the psychogeriatrician.
> No dementia, Loretta thinks, almost weightless with the joy of it.

***

The second psychiatrist I saw was the one that calmed my anxiety over my visions. This was after seeing a GP, another psychiatrist, an ophthalmologist, a retinal specialist, and a psychologist.

"Normal", he says. "Charles Bonnet syndrome, but it's not at all uncommon for people losing sight to have these visions".

So, there's a simple explanation for these complex visual hallucinations, but it took a while to get there. So much worry for so long.

Charles Bonnet syndrome

The syndrome of vivid visual hallucinations occurring for people with low vision is named after Charles Bonnet. These hallucinations tend to be recurrent. You'll note that visual hallucinations can occur in other conditions that affect older people such as

Parkinson's disease and dementia. But here we're focusing on the visual hallucinations that occur in people with conditions producing low vision.

Charles Bonnet (1720–1793) was a Swiss scholar. His grandfather, Charles Lullin, had advanced cataracts and vision loss. Lullin kept a diary describing in detail his visual hallucinations as they came and went. Bonnet himself was partially deaf since childhood, suffered progressive vision loss from his twenties, and visual hallucinations like his grandfather, in middle age. Bonnet was a renowned scientist, becoming a fellow of the French Academy of Sciences at 20 after an article on reproduction, without sperm, of the female aphid tree lice. Membership of the Royal College in London followed, after a treatise on the function of plant leaves. But as he aged, he could no longer use microscopes, relying on assistants for his research as his eyesight worsened. In 1760, Charles Bonnet wrote *Analytical Essays on Concerning the Faculties of the Mind* (or the Soul depending on the translation of *l'Ame*) in which he described the visual hallucinations or "fictions of the brain" that his 90 year old grandfather has diarized in detail, writing:

> …I should tell about a strange case that would be considered fabulous if not supported by testimonies of the highest credibility…I will simply say that I know a respectable man full of health, of ingenuousness, judgement, and memory, who, completely alert and independently from all outside influences, sees from time to time, in front of him, figures of men, of women, of birds, of carriages, of buildings et. …. All these visions appear

to him in perfect clarity and affect him as strongly as if as the objects themselves were present.

(Hedges, 2007, p. 112)

This establishes the features of what Georges de Morsier, a French physician in 1936 called Charles Bonnet syndrome. At first, he believed that vision loss was not a prerequisite and by 1967, this was amended. This marked the start of diagnostic uncertainty with a split between disciplines where neurologists favor definitions with visual hallucinations in patients with and without low vision; but ophthalmologists apply the classic 1760 triad: patients with low vision, no cognitive or mental illness experiencing simple or complex recurring visual hallucinations.

While a variety of realistic illusions may appear, they may be simple (for instance, flashes) or complex (people, landscapes, objects etc.); they are not accompanied by sound effects. Bonnet ascribed the origin of these phantasms as "in the part of the brain that commands the sense of sight" (Hedges, 2007, p. 113). So, his reasoning was that the brain of a person losing their sight (and therefore deprived of visual stimuli) emits visual images where there are none to be seen. Lullins'"playthings of the mind" began in later old age, and Bonnet's own phantasms began in his forties when he retired to his estates in Genthod, Switzerland. Here, he also dictated eight volumes of *Works of Natural History and Philosophy* (*Œuvres d'histoire naturelle et de philosophie*) to his secretary.

As mentioned, Bonnet adjusted his career to his low vision. The visual hallucinations he experienced did not impede his progress in this major scientific undertaking. He also had the comfort of knowing, from his observations of his grandfather's spectacu-lar spectrals that no harm or cognitive decline would accom-pany them.

Such knowledge is limited for the rest of us: Loretta and I simply didn't know, despite my medical degree and work, and Loretta's nursing studies and long nursing career. There are many case examples and cautionary tales in the literature about the havoc that these hallucinations wreak: people diagnosed with mental illnesses they don't have, because the visions are seen as evidence of psychosis or dementia. Those seeing the unseen can end up in psychiatric institutions or residential aged care and are believed to have diminished capacity for self-care and determination.

So, Charles Bonnet syndrome, as we understand it, relates to peo-ple living with low vision, hallucinations, and intact cognition; but it was not until recent decades that there has been more research interest in the syndrome. Jones et al. (2021) reports that examining the database PubMed demonstrates an increasing trajectory in publications that relate to CBS, with almost two thirds published papers in the last 10 years.

We still don't know *exactly* what causes the phenomena and we don't know *exactly* how common it is; lack of awareness and the presence of stigma means that doctors underdiagnose and patients underreport these symptoms. We do know however, that visual hallucinations cause problems for many who live with the hidden fear of psychiatric or neurodegenerative conditions, who may struggle with quality of life with disruptions to sleep, education, and work (Jones et al., 2021). We also understand that some people with low vision are more at risk of developing the syndrome than others. Known risk factors include increased age, social isolation, low cognitive function, history of stroke, and poor bilateral visual acuity (Nair et al., 2015). Pang (2016) also notes that the incidence is higher in people with dual sensory impairment (DSI) than those with low vision only. So, hearing loss combined with vision loss has some sort of additive impact that we don't yet fully understand.

And it also seems that stressful life events and natural disasters can precipitate or worsen hallucinations in at risk individuals (Jones et al., 2021; Vucicevik, 2010).

Now, we will provide a brief overview of the characteristics and management of Charles Bonnet syndrome to raise awareness among the public and professionals.

Common causes of vision loss

There is no exhaustive list available of all the possible causes of vision loss in those with the syndrome. Age-related macular degeneration, glaucoma, and cataracts are the three most common causes of vision loss noted in those with Charles Bonnet syndrome (Nair et al., 2015.

Basically however, if a condition can cause vision loss, a person can experience visual hallucinations.

Nature and form of visual hallucinations

The hallucinations experienced in Charles Bonnet syndrome are many and varied; they can be formed or unformed, simple or complex, in full color or black and white, moving or stationary.

Episodes usually last seconds to minutes. The hallucinations can be distressing and disruptive. Sleep can be affected. For another lived experience account see Nieman (2018), in which a doctor, describes his hallucinations, their form, and impact.

Around three quarters of those with Charles Bonnet syndrome may eventually accept the hallucinations as part of a "new normal" life with low vision. But for many the "silent doubt" of "am I insane" lingers (Lopes and Sales, 2016, p. s471).

Simple hallucinations can include the already mentioned flashes and also lights (sometimes called photopsia), dots, shapes, or tessellopsia (patterns like tiles). It is thought some 41–59 percent of those with low vision experience the simple type (Kennard, 2018). Complex hallucinations are experienced by 11–15 percent (Kennard, 2018). These involve objects, faces (familiar or unfamiliar), figures (adults, children, dressed, undressed), animals, insects (butterflies and caterpillars for example), surfaces, textures, rooms, and landscapes. Images may be realistic, or grotesque and deformed. As indicated earlier, oscillopsia, also known as movement, may be present, such as people moving down hallways, in and out of houses, around beds (Nair et al., 2015). Dr. Nieman describes his own hallucinations of text written on top of fog (Nieman, 2018).

There may be cultural and religious aspects to complex hallucinations such as seeing religious deities. Nair et al. (2015) report that in India where religion is an integral part of life, hallucinations involving religious figures may be viewed by the hallucinators and their caregivers as "divine interactions". Patients may be comforted or terrified by religious or profane apparitions.

Other authors such as Das et al. (2020) and Buyukgol et al. (2018) note that Indian and Turkish patients respectively, are less likely to report hallucinations because of the cultural stigma and fear associated with a perceived mental health diagnosis. Similarly, a Danish study reported over 60 percent of those living with visual hallucinations experienced fear of being labeled "insane" if they disclosed these hallucinations (Menon, 2005). Most of the works cited here note that these beliefs are widespread among most patient groups (and exemplified in the account by Loretta and I). The patient, and often family held fears are compounded by the prevailing lack of patient, health professional, and community awareness of the syndrome. And sometimes, unfortunately, medical practitioners perpetuate the misbeliefs with erroneous diagnoses, treatments, and even institutionalization.

Generally, it seems most people over time come to feel impartial about their hallucinations with one study putting this figure at 70 percent. Five percent report experiencing hallucinations as pleasant.

However, approximately 25 percent felt their visual hallucinations were unpleasant or distressing (Kahn et al., 2008). For many, the hallucinations worsen as the day progresses. One type of complex hallucination that is often associated with distress is prosopometamorphopsia, which is when facial features become grossly distorted (Jones et al., 2021). An example of this is Loretta's description of the little girl in the red coat's face.

The duration of Charles Bonnet syndrome was originally thought to be short, of less than 18 months (Kennard, 2018). But we now realize (and as evidenced above in the lived experience accounts and some studies) that hallucinations may last longer than five years.

Finally, it is important to stress that hallucinations are not always static, identical, or singular for an individual. They may change over time, from simple to complex; additional hallucinations may occur such as in my case with the phantasmic watch face as well as the man in the dark suit. Jones et al. (2021) notes, "The reports suggest that more extensive visual loss is associated with more complex and enduring hallucinations". On the other hand, regression and cessation of hallucinations as vision becomes severely or totally limited is also well noted. External events and life stressors may precipitate or amplify visual hallucinations, (for example, being evacuated from a deadly bushfire in one case report resulted in worsening hallucinations) (Vucicevik, 2010).

The Covid pandemic of 2020 to present has also been considered a stressor event with loneliness and isolation precipitating or worsening visual hallucinations in patients with low vision (Jones et al., 2021).

Conversely, patients with Charles Bonnet syndrome and loneliness/social isolation may report temporary amelioration of symptoms when in hospital (for other causes) and receiving care and communication (Menon et al., 2003).

Causal mechanisms

There are many theories as to the causal mechanism of the syndrome. At present, the most accepted is "deafferentation" whereby increased activity in the visual cortex occurs following reduced sensory input from the eyes (Jones et al., 2021; Kennard,

2018). Some have likened the visual hallucinations to phantom limb pain: "Severe vision impairment (and decreased visual stimuli) leads to the production of *de novo* images from the visual cortex causing visual hallucinations (Nair et al., 2015). Another putative mechanism is the neuromatrix theory, which posits that throughout the brain a network of neurons, called the neuromatrix, can spontaneously produce visual phenomena experienced as hallucinations (Das et al., 2020; Nair et al., 2015). The lack of a solid mechanism of causation has implications for treatments when needed for refractory and distressing hallucinations as no single drug therapy has been found to consistently ameliorate the condition.

How common is the syndrome?

The data around the prevalence of Charles Bonnet syndrome are imprecise, principally due to the already mentioned underdiagnosis by doctors and underreporting by patients. While some early studies suggest that approximately 11–15 percent of patients with vision loss experience visual hallucinations, Niazi et al. (2020), in a systematic review of the syndrome in patients with age-related macular degeneration, put the figure at 31.6 percent. Baldock et al. (2017) found a rate of 35 percent in healthy older adults experiencing vision loss. We have been unable to find data for the syndrome's prevalence in patients with DSI, but Pang (2016) noted that visual hallucinations are "more common" in patients with DSI. This makes sense given the very high rates of hearing loss in older people generally. Many of those with the syndrome must also have hearing loss. This can add complexity, as the fear and anxiety generated in the hallucinatory experience may worsen social coping, and so promote social isolation, which in turn may increase the hallucinations. Those providing clinical care and support to patients with Charles Bonnet syndrome (and those with low vision with and without hearing loss more broadly) need to be aware of the role social isolation/loneliness may play in the precipitation and perpetuation of visual hallucinations. One study suggested loneliness—in the sense of poor quality of social relationships, rather than simply the number of social contacts—may be associated with the syndrome (Jones et al., 2021). Browning discusses this more broadly when she states: "people with dual sensory impairment don't need **more** social contact, they need better communication quality in the ones they want to have" (DUAL-SIG meeting, November, 2022). These observations point to the need to support patients with low vision and hearing loss more wholistically, with a team knowledgeable about DSI and Charles Bonnet syndrome.

We also don't know much about multi modal hallucinations generally and more specifically in older people with low vision and/or hearing loss. And little is known about the relationship between auditory hallucinations, for example, that occur separately to Charles Bonnet syndrome. People with hearing loss can "hear" voices and other sounds in much the same way, but these don't have a visual accompaniment (see Oliver Sacks for further detail). Tinnitus is very common in older people however, and we discuss this shortly.

Clinical challenges

There are many challenges for health and social care professionals in the diagnosis and support of those living with visual hallucinations. Firstly, there exists no consensus on a definition of Charles Bonnet syndrome, and not withstanding this there are low levels of awareness among clinicians, patients, and the community (Pang, 2016). Diagnosis is complicated because it requires cross-disciplinary assessments. Patients are hesitant to seek medical advice, as discussed earlier. Treatments are complicated by the absence of guidelines and large-scale clinical studies. This leaves health professional knowledge dependent on case reports and small studies on a wide variety of medications, none of which reliably eliminates hallucinations in most patients (Jones et al., 2021; Pang, 2016).

A Canadian study by Gordan and Felfeli (2018) reports a low level of syndrome knowledge among general practitioners/ family physicians. No awareness at all was shown by 55 percent and 85 percent never discussed visual hallucinations with their patients presenting with low vision.

Worryingly, some patients too, feel their treating professionals lack knowledge of the syndrome (Cox and Ffytche, 2014). Austrian research by Doeller et al. (2021) demonstrates that patients benefit from explanations and reassurance from professionals who are knowledgeable about the syndrome. In Australia, the Charles Bonnet Syndrome Foundation is working with the Royal Australian College of General Practitioners to promote awareness among GPs there (Charles Bonnet Syndrome Foundation, 2023).

As stated, low levels of community and patient awareness means low rates of help-seeking and high rates of anxiety and fear in people (and families/carers) experiencing visual hallucinations. A Danish specialist eye clinic revealed knowledge about the syndrome was sparse with only 12 percent of patients attending the clinic being aware of the syndrome. Among the 88 percent who were unaware of the syndrome, 13.1 percent were found to experience visual hallucinations (Singh, Subhi and Sørensen, 2014). This again demonstrates the failure of medical professionals to be aware and knowledgeable and reinforces the need to educate patients with low vision before the potential onset of hallucinations.

Belonging to a support organization is likely to improve awareness, for example Cox and Ffytche (2014) report almost 90 percent of the members of the Macular Society in the UK were knowledgeable about the syndrome.

Other diagnostic challenges are aplenty. Visual hallucinations have a broad differential diagnosis and may present across a wide range of clinical disciplines. So, misdiagnosis is not uncommon. Alongside underdiagnosis and underreporting of the syndrome generally is the simple fact that a great number of people experience *elementary visual phenomena* such as flashes, lights, shapes, and dots. Flashes and floaters are very common as we age as the vitreous (gel like substance in the eye) shrinks, liquefies, and detaches from the wall of the inner eye. So, many of the simple hallucinations may be disregarded as being symptomatic only of advancing age.

Some with the syndrome are misdiagnosed with other ocular pathologies, e.g., retinal tears and detachment with the onset of flashing lights or floaters (photopsia). What this means in practice is that a great deal of care and time should go into history taking (ask patients if they are experiencing any unusual "sights"), examination, and testing before pronouncing diagnoses or dismissing concerns.

Another diagnostic issue is the classic diagnostic triad requiring intact cognition with the experience of visual hallucinations and ocular pathology. Does this mean people with dementia never get Charles Bonnet syndrome? Or does it mean it is "too hard" to disentangle the causation as dementia and neurodegenerative conditions are associated with visual hallucinations without, as well as with, ocular pathologies? Do we even need to disentangle causations? The Study of Hallucinations in Parkinson's Disease, Eye Disease and Dementia (SHAPED) (Ffytche et al., 2017) is examining diagnosis and two treatment options in those three conditions. This may result in some progress in discriminating visual hallucinations in different conditions where eye disease is present (or not).

Management

Here, we sketch a roadmap to better recognize and support those living with or at risk of experiencing visual hallucinations of Charles Bonnet syndrome. Management needs to begin prior to the onset of hallucinations by informing all those with low vision about the syndrome and its largely benign nature.

Management roadmap for Charles Bonnet syndrome: List 1

1.   Educating professionals
     Undergraduate, postgraduate, and continuing professional development for medical, nursing, allied health, specialists, ophthalmologists, optometrists, psychogeriatricians,

geriatricians, rehabilitation clinicians, audiologists, ear nose and throat surgeons, head and neck surgeons and neurologists, aged care workers, social care practitioners. All need to become syndrome aware.

2.   Raising community awareness

Professionals and support organizations to provide all people with low vision with education about Charles Bonnet syndrome before the possible onset of hallucinations.

3.   Forewarning patients at risk (and their families)

4.   Reassurance and explanations

Professionals to: ask, listen, investigate, diagnose, provide reassurance, and explanations to the patient and family of the largely benign nature.

5.   Use diagnostic tools as an adjunct to clinical assessment, e.g., QR-SCB

The French-language Questionnaire de repérage du syndromede Charles Bonnet (QR-SCB); in English, Charles Bonnet Syndrome Screening Questionnaire aims to identify the syndrome and locate those patients who need further intervention (see Cantin et al., 2019).

6.   Provide referrals to support services and organizations

Referral to support groups, for example www.charlesbon netsyndrome.uk and www.charlesbonnetsyndrome.org

7.   Behavioral strategies

Suggestions include frequent blinking or rapid eye movements or changing the light levels to increase visual input and alerting/distraction techniques (Jones et al., 2021). Exercise, reading, listening to music, changing a person's physical environment have also been found helpful to some.

8. Counseling

    Should be offered to all because living with vision loss generally is associated with higher rates of psychoemotional distress, and living with visual hallucinations can be a source of great anxiety and distress.

    Extra support may be needed in times of high stress given that these may precipitate, increase, or alter the nature of hallucinations.

9. Carer support

    Carer burden is often and invisible, (see Chapter 5). Physical, psychological, and respite services may be needed.

10. Optimization of vision

    Treat the underlying cause of low vision where possible, e.g., remove cataracts. This is especially important in the developing world where low vision due to cataracts is especially high.

11. Support better living with low vision

    Orientation and mobility training, aids, and accommodations.

    Stimulate the senses with exercise, walks, reading, music, audiobooks, social engagement with others, puzzles, and games.

    Promotion of better quality social encounters.

12. Pharmacotherapies

    Considered in refractory cases where hallucinations are causing disruption and distress. There are no evidenced-based guidelines we could find but "trial and error" possibilities include: antipsychotics, anticonvulsants, anxiolytics, and antidepressants.

13. Collaboration

Well informed teams of professionals caring for patients with the syndrome make a difference to coping resilience and outcomes (Jones et al., 2021).

14. Fund, foster, and participate in research

Grow the body of knowledge about visual hallucinations in people with low vision. In particular, invest in lived experience qualitative research to generate knowledge from those expert-knowers living with DSI and Charles Bonnet syndrome.

Tinnitus
Hearing the unheard: DSI and tinnitus

You don't have to live with DSI to experience tinnitus. Author one notes "last night I got bad tinnitus: there was a tap tap tap tapping that went on for hours. It was irritating as I was trying to sleep. I knew what it was and ended up reading to distract myself and eventually fell asleep. I often 'hear the unheard', and hearing aids do sometimes mask the noises by blasting other ones over the top. But nothing other the passing of time, be it minutes, hours or half a night, sees the end of an episode".

In addition to those with DSI "seeing the unseen", we are also aware that those with DSI may also experience "hearing the unheard" in the form of phantom auditory sounds that can vary in intensity, duration, and the level of impact on a persons' life. This is known as tinnitus and is commonly associated with hearing loss. The word "tinnitus" comes from the Latin verb *tinnere*, meaning to ring. But people may experience simple ringing, buzzing, hissing, crackling, humming, and more. Less common are complex sounds such as voices, telephones, doorbells. Sounds may be high pitched or low, they may be soft or loud. They may be tolerable to very disruptive.

The heterogeneity and subjectivity of tinnitus make it particularly challenging to research, manage, and provide specific services to those who experience it. Despite its prevalence, there are few treatment options and most are directed at reducing the personal impact of the condition (McFerran et al., 2019).

Tinnitus is an "invisible", common, and often debilitating experience which refers to the perception of sound in the absence of any external stimuli (Baguley et al., 2013; Gopinath et al., 2013). Commonly referred to as "ringing in the ears", tinnitus is estimated to affect 10–15 percent of adults worldwide, can occur across the lifespan, but increases with age (Baguley et al., 2013; Henry et al., 2020; Bauer, 2018), with prevalence estimates of 30 percent in those over 55 years (Newall et al., 2001). Definitions and diagnostic criteria for tinnitus differ internationally meaning that there is widespread variability in prevalence estimates (McCormack et al., 2016). Tinnitus can be subjective and individually based; or objective, where the stimulus can be heard externally (much less common) (Baguley et al., 2013). Here we focus on the subjective experience of tinnitus. Henry et al. (2020) suggest that a clear definition is critical; this should distinguish specific tinnitus characteristics such as timing, constancy, and degree of emotional and physical impact on day-to-day living.

There is little research on the association of DSI with tinnitus although given that age-related hearing loss is strongly associated with tinnitus, it makes sense that of those with DSI, a proportion may also experience tinnitus.

Risk factors

There are a number of known risk factors for tinnitus: the degree of hearing loss, overall general health (including factors such as smoking and alcohol), impaired cardiovascular and cerebrovascular function, and exposure over lifetime to both occupational and non-occupational noise (Henry et al., 2020). It is noted in several studies that military veterans have a higher overall risk of developing chronic tinnitus than non-veterans (Hoffman and Reed, 2004; Moring et al., 2018; Theodoroff et al., 2015). Further information on military veterans and tinnitus and hearing loss can be found in the following current longitudinal study, Noise Outcomes in Service Members Epidemiology Study (NOISE study). Others such as Baguley et al. (2013, p. 484) noted co-morbidities such as depression, anxiety, temporomandibular joint disorder (TMJ), and hyperacusis.

Impacts

Tinnitus is a symptom, such as pain, and not an illness. The person with the tinnitus is the only one who can describe what they hear and how disturbing it is for them. For most people, the perception of tinnitus gets better over time. The impacts of tinnitus vary depending on the severity experienced. Quality of life can be significantly impacted and there is a lack of lived experience voices in current research. There are some exceptions to this: Zarenoe and Ledin's, (2014) study explored quality of life in patients with tinnitus in Sweden, with just under half the sample (46%, n=175 participants) describing treatment as "not good" or absent. Others, such as McFerron et al. (2019, p. 2) investigated patient experiences of tinnitus services and management in the UK and found that while diagnostic strategies were considered appropriate, the ongoing management of tinnitus was "unsatisfactory". Overall, there was a mismatch between patient and audiologist expectations with audiologists focused on management, and patients on "cure".

The impacts can be debilitating on a day-to-day basis with those experiencing severe tinnitus reporting headaches, insomnia, poor concentration, and reduced socialization, leading to stress and isolation (Durai et al., 2017). Tinnitus is also associated with anxiety and depression; in a recent systematic review of 28 international studies, Salazar et al. (2019) noted the median prevalence for depression was 33 percent.

Family and carers

Similar to DSI research, there is little research exploring the impact and experiences of tinnitus on family members, or third party disability. Third party disability is the experience of negative consequences as a result of their family members' chronic health issue or disability (Scarinci et al., 2009), and these indirect effects impact relationships and social activities. Beukes et al. (2022) qualitative analysis of the significant others of those with tinnitus, noted the social, relational, and emotional toll experienced by these significant others. One participant in this study identified a reduction in social activities:

> Our social life and time with our adult kids has been
> affected as well. When we are in a big family gathering,
> he will leave the room because he gets so anxious over
> the noise level. It is embarrassing. Or I go to the func-
> tions without him, which sucks.
>
> (Beukes et al., 2022)

And, despite modifications to their lifestyle, a number of significant others in this study also reported feeling helpless and sad
(p. 7). Mancini et al. (2019) notes a disconnect between persons
with tinnitus and their significant others or communication
partners in terms of their understanding of the condition itself,
and how it impacts each of them; there was a lack of discussion
around tinnitus and a lack of clarity on how best to support their
significant other with tinnitus.

Management

A family and person-centered approach to managing tinnitus
(with or without DSI) that includes psychological, emotional, and
social support for both those with tinnitus *and* their family, is
important to managing the day-to-day impact of tinnitus, with
or without DSI.

Other key strategies for managing tinnitus are very similar to
those for Charles Bonnet syndrome:

- Medical and audiology review: maintaining good overall
  health including control of high blood pressure and a medical check are recommended. Discussion with an audiologist
  on the perception and experience of tinnitus. The audiologist may be able to provide tinnitus-acclimatization therapy,
  recommend sound devices, or adjust your own hearing aids

to help reduce the perception of the tinnitus. Listening to music or watching television may also help some;

- Raising awareness among individuals with sensory loss/es, carers and families, community;
- Increasing knowledge of health and social care professionals about lived experience of tinnitus and its impacts;
- Exploring contributing factors such as vitamin B12 deficiency, medication side effects, e.g., high dose aspirin, alcohol and caffeine, cardiovascular and cerebrovascular disease;
- Some tinnitus can be triggered or amplified by tension in the head and neck area, including the jaws. Addressing potential tensions in these areas with a physiotherapist or a dentist can provide relief;
- Strategies such as massage of the neck, ears, tempomandibular region can help lower general stress levels and reduce tension in the head and neck for some;
- Sound therapy devices including hearing aids, as introducing more ambient noise can mask the tinnitus thereby decreasing its impact on the individual;
- Behavioral strategies such as reducing alcohol and caffeine intake, improved sleep hygiene;
- Psychological strategies including stress reduction measures, mindfulness, cognitive behavioral therapy aimed at habituation and coping;
- Natural therapies such as acupuncture have been shown to be effective for some and may be useful in removing tension in the head and neck area, and decreasing general stress levels;
- Medications/pharmacotherapy such as antidepressants, anxiolytics, anticonvulsants can be helpful for a few of those

experiencing disruptive symptoms. However, it must be stressed that there is very limited evidence or guidelines for these treatments. Most must be prescribed "off label". No treatment exists or is FDA, Therapeutic Goods Administration (TGA) of Australia approved, for tinnitus that is curative or effective for all or most who experience the condition;

• Explore new innovations such as Lenire, approved by the US Food and Drug Administration as a non-invasive neuro-modulation device to minimize tinnitus in 2023. This device combines auditory and electrical stimuli to diminish the experience of tinnitus. Further studies are needed; and

• Greater investment in lived experience research and increasing treatment options.

Summary

Tinnitus is likely to impact those with DSI, and potentially add greater complexity to the delivery of appropriate support and services. Similar to the DSI narrative, there are challenges in the heterogeneity of tinnitus; the lack of treatment options and clear understanding of the condition itself, and its impacts (both public and health professionals). All these factors present challenges for health professionals when managing clients with tinnitus, or tinnitus *and* DSI.

In Australia, there are a number of resources that provide support and education. These are listed below:

• Health Direct, Tinnitus, Australian Government

• The Tinnitus Australia Roadmap https://tinnitusaustralia.org.au/the-tinnitus-australia-roadmap/

• Roadmap for Hearing Health, Australian Government Department of Health and Aged Care

Health professionals can also direct clients to the following client focused resources:

1.   www.mindear.com/solution
2.   https://tinnitusaustralia.org.au/supporting-you/

5
The effort and art of caring

Introduction

So far, we have explored the complex intersectional issues that limit access, increase social isolation, and threaten health and well-being for older adults with dual sensory impairment (DSI). This chapter now looks at family carers specifically and how they describe their experiences of living with an older person with DSI; these are sometimes described as "informal carers". We look too at the strategies they use to manage and confront the many complexities. We will see that the invisible epidemic of rising numbers of older adults with DSI extends also to an intensifying carer burden. This chapter provides an overview of caring in Australia more broadly before focusing on the key aspects of caring in a DSI context.

Caring in Australia

Most advanced economies embrace the notion of "aging in place", upholding the decision making and rights of older adults to remain at home in older age, often despite complex age-related health problems (Kendig et al., 2017; Pani-Harreman et al., 2021; Pavey et al., 2009). To support these decisions, care needs are often supported by a combination of informal and formal (government-funded) care (AIHW, 2021b). The terminology "family carers" and "informal carers" is used interchangeably to describe the care delivered to support the needs of older persons "aging in place"; for the purposes of this text, we will use the term "family carers". These mixed care networks are integral to the continued functioning of health systems. Family carers provide most of the care to those at home, including the older person, with an estimated 2.65 million (unpaid) informal carers in Australia in 2018 (ABS, 2018). The World Health Organization estimates that informal caring subsidizes healthcare systems to approximately 3.6 percent of GDP in Europe, while a Deloitte report in 2020 estimated the cost of replacing all informal caring in Australia at **77.9 billion** (Deloitte Access Economics, 2020); this suggests that care in this context has valuable cost benefit impacts to system funding. With informal caring in Australia (see Australian Institute of Health and Welfare for definitions of carers) considered an integral part of the Australian healthcare landscape from a cost benefit perspective, there is now increasing attention directed to the impacts of caring and carers' needs (Eagar et al., 2007; Kelley et al., 2017; ABS, 2018, as the physically and mentally arduous nature of caring suggests that the demand of a rapidly aging population will increasingly outstrip supply (Deloitte Access Economics, 2020; Eagar et al., 2007; Shu et al., 2019).

Formal versus informal caring

With over half of the population in Australia aged over 65 years living with disability and complex age-related health issues (ABS,

2020), the proportion of this population who may require care or rely on support networks is growing (AIHW, 2021a). Aged-care policies and legislation that preference home care over residential care (e.g., Aged Care (Living Longer Living Better) Act, (Cth), 2013; Moore, 2021) have seen the growth of informal caring for older Australians living with a range of health needs. In Australia, formal carers are defined as those who are funded by the Australian Government and provide specific care to those eligible and living at home or in the community (ABS, 2020). Informal carers are most often family members and more likely to be female (12.3% of all females) than male (9.3% of all males) (ABS, 2020b).

Caring in a DSI context

In the context of DSI, Senses Australia reports that almost 80 percent of those aged over 60 years with DSI live at home, and for those aged over 85 years, assistance is required for at least one activity (Dyke, 2013). Additionally, 82 percent of those aged over 60 years report requiring assistance from a family carer (p. 54). While informal caring in Australia is now considered fundamental to the Australian healthcare landscape (Eagar et al., 2007), integrating a complex network of support that blends formal and informal care is necessary, in order to support both carers and care receivers (Cleary et al., 2006). Although this suggests that a network of support may provide the best "fit" for those with DSI, there are a number of reasons suggesting that this may not happen: i) The previously noted reduction in social interaction of the person with DSI may limit opportunities to engage with family or government agencies to seek the support needed; ii) Poor recognition of DSI by both family and person with DSI means that a specific need is not met; and iii) Carers recognize the caring needs of their family member with DSI but may not understand the root cause of these needs. As has been noted in previous chapters, the lack of legislative recognition of distinct disability status and poor community and professional recognition of DSI, increase carer burden; additionally, even when DSI is recognized, specific DSI services are relatively non-existent.

There is limited research on the impacts of caring in a DSI context specifically. The conflation of aging with DSI means that separating DSI as the root cause for caring needs is complex, often existing on a background of age-related ill-health for both carer and care receiver (person with DSI). The lack of DSI visibility *and* specific strategies aligned to the older person with DSI more broadly, limits understanding at micro, meso and macro levels. While current research on the caring role in a DSI context remains limited, authors, such as Lehane et al. (2017, 2018) and Hofsöe et al. (2019) suggest that understanding DSI from a collective perspective has potential to offer a more nuanced and targeted approach that may enhance quality of life for both. As such, we see the impacts of DSI as a shared experience. The findings from Dunsmore (2022) support the shared experience of DSI and is considered in the sections to follow: i) The effort of caring and; ii) The art of caring.

The effort of caring in a DSI context

As the consequences of DSI are often intangible, those with DSI may not meet the criteria for additional support through formal aged care despite often experiencing significant functional impairment. Most often, caring needs are met by family car-ers who take on multiple roles which range from support with activities of daily living through to social and emotional care. This carer role, despite the multiplicity of responsibilities, lacks visibility and recognition, which has consequences for the carer relationship in terms of public awareness, and therefore public empathy. As noted, DSI may exist for a period of time prior to recognition (if recognized at all) so the adoption of a caregiv-ing role, particularly for spousal carers, can impact an already strained relationship, often on a background of age-related ill-health of the carer themselves. Intermittent and a "give and take" type of reciprocal caregiving is typical of many family relation-ships, particularly in managing chronic health issues, such as sensory losses. In aging, this can transition to a more permanent caregiving role, which necessitates changes to well-established roles and responsibilities within the family unit (Carpenter and Mak, 2007; Monin et al., 2019). This can impact the identity and perception of personal autonomy for the family caregiver (Wallhagen, 1993).

A dyad refers to two persons in a relationship existing over a long period of time, that leads to interdependence (Barnes, 2015). The caregiving dyad is made up of the person with DSI and their family carer (often spouse, daughter, son). This is the simplest deconstruction of a more complex social network and is criti-cal to healthy aging. The family carer can provide social support and facilitate social engagement for the care receiver; however, they also play a complex role in accessing external social sup-ports and resources for their family member. The increased social effort required for this can place additional strain on the existing relationship and create significant interpersonal tension, and health impacts for the family carer. There is limited research to date on this.

Social isolation and effort

Family carers provide day-to-day support for their family member in terms of navigating public spaces, including the healthcare system, and managing activities of daily living. There is significant and often unrecognized effort in this support. There is recognition of the need to remain socially engaged (for both), but this is increasingly difficult due to safety concerns and social disengagement when in social situations. Multiple and ongoing missed social opportunities create resentment and exacerbate interpersonal tension, often due to a mismatch of expectations and needs of caregiver and care receiver. Much of this is related to misunderstanding of DSI and the perception that those with DSI could "try harder" as they are not "fully blind and deaf" (family carers' narratives, Dunsmore, 2022). This lack of understanding is more broadly pervasive: DSI as a spectrum underscores the need for person-centered care and a focus on the individual rather than the broad "one size fits all" approach which is common in healthcare.

Social difficulties exist at the interpersonal level (between family carer and person with DSI), and more broadly at social events. Missed communication and fractured conversations contribute to embarrassing social encounters and despite carers' understanding of the need to engage socially, the effort required often outweighs the benefits. This highlights the fact that living with DSI means receiving information in fragments (see Nordic definition, Chapter 2). In social (and other) circumstances, family and friends have to modify their communication:

> You have to basically modify your whole way of com-
> municating, its like being in a foreign country and you
> have to…more or less think that the other person is….
> not able to understand you, so it is a constant strain.
>
> (Carer)

There is effort also in "sharing the story" of DSI during social encounters. The lack of visible signs of disability mean that family carers adopt a protective role in managing others' social expectations, including explaining DSI, time and again, contributing to the communication fatigue family carers experience. There is recognition of the complexities of social interactions with many family carers feeling the need to intervene on their family members behalf to maintain social conversation. Communication tension is common with family carers on constant alert to interpret social cues on behalf of their family member; their role as social facilitator is constant, often subtle, and tiring.

Social effort and communication fatigue extends to healthcare interactions, both within the hospital setting and in primary care, especially at GP visits. Healthcare encounters increase in frequency with age and many carers describe these encounters as frustrating and negative. We know that DSI is underreported in healthcare and poorly acknowledged in health policy development (Dullard and Saunders, 2016; Jaiswal et al., 2018) which undermines the autonomy of those with DSI in healthcare settings and makes essential the need for accompaniment to these settings. Poor attitudes, low awareness, and inattention to communication needs from health caregivers can contribute to poor experiences and adverse outcomes (see Chapter 3). Additionally, family carers in this study (Dunsmore, 2022) described interactions in primary care where the effects of DSI were minimized:

> There's another thing too about the GP, the sort of mentality 'Well what do you expect? You're 95'. These days we're all harping on about people with disabilities and how they have to be accommodated, but hearing and vision loss in old age is not seen as a disability, it's seen as something else.
>
> (Sarah)

These issues underscore the dependence of those with DSI on their family carer to navigate systems, communicate their needs, and advocate for them. Of course, this also highlights potential privacy concerns and the potential for missed health information. Greater attention by healthcare professionals to effective communication strategies may help decrease carer burden here.

Changing roles

Family carers made significant effort to navigate their changing circumstances, often with little understanding of the cause of their increasing responsibilities and need for change. Their caring role did not easily fit with the social norm of caring and many carers found it difficult to articulate the social aspects of their caring role. The increasing dependence of their family member, the number of missed social opportunities for both, and the lack of explicit diagnosis and support structures available meant that family carers shared the impacts of DSI, becoming increasingly isolated and with little time for anything else. This highlights in Australia, how the lack of recognition of DSI as a unique and distinct disability, an absence in policy and planning, and negligible dedicated support services has profound negative consequences for the dyad. This broad whole-of-society lack of understanding of DSI meant that finding more formalized care for the person with DSI can be limited; additionally, the specific communication needs of DSI meant that government-funded formal carers were ill-equipped to manage the needs of older persons with DSI. Additionally, sourcing appropriate and specific formal support can be difficult for family carers, with government-funded service provision for care of older persons in the community acknowledged as low-paid and insecure, with little specific communication training for supporting those with DSI. Family carers in Dunsmore (2022), described communication difficulties with these carers and the lack of choice and consistency in carer provision from the aged-care package (Australian Government, 2020). This means that both members of the caring dyad were reluctant to engage in this form of external care:

> It needs to be someone who speaks reasonably good English, and there aren't any…it's got to be people who are able to put the time and effort into building that rapport and all that kind of thing.
>
> (Carer)

Family carers changing roles were characterized by shrinking networks, missed opportunities, and isolation from their own networks. The effort of caring reflects the lack of clarity family carers experienced in understanding their role, shaped by preconceptions of a more "traditional" caring role where physical needs were more obvious. Instead, caring in a DSI context was predominantly social, often intangible, and complex to articulate to others. The absence of guidance or acknowledgment of their role intensified the sense of invisibility experienced by family carers, impacted their relationships, and compounded the social isolation experienced by both.

We also acknowledge here that caring roles in older age may be interchangeable; those with DSI may be family carers themselves which adds another layer of complexity (Simcock, 2017; Watharow, 2021).

In Chapter 1, we heard from Victor who embodies multi-layered caring roles. Victor is an older adult with DSI, and the carer for his wife/partner who has multiple disabilities, including DSI. He is also invested in welfare checks in his poorly managed residential aged-care facility. Victor has bilateral optic atrophy and hearing loss from occupational noise exposure. He wears hearing aids and loves it when others don't realize he is also blind! His wife Mabel has DSI as well as numerous other health conditions and is often in hospital. Since their families did not want to live with them, they moved into a "home" where there's no accommodation for a married couple, so Victor and Mabel have rooms 25 meters apart in the facility.

Victor says, "It's a bit like living on Mars since Covid, with all the gear, masks, shields, and gowns. Sometimes in an outbreak we are just stuck in our rooms for days and weeks and even months, no one looking in or helping or anything". Victor compensates supporting other residents with advocacy and supervision, "I'm the only one here able to do things. The rest are all too sick or too old to do anything". Victor and Mabel describe management as neglectful, "Everyone here is old and has disabilities…. It is isolating…I've found three people dead here—I've got it going that if you haven't seen your neighbor…we need to know about it".

As well, Victor is committed to supporting his wife not only at home but also in hospital. He says, "Getting information is the hardest part…so I have learned to just go to the nurses' station and stay there until someone tells me what I need to know about Mabel".

The art of caring: Rethinking caring in a DSI context

As previously noted, family carers play a crucial role in facilitating social interaction and navigating healthcare for their family member with DSI. The perceived effort of this appears, at least in part, dependent on the carer's level of empathic understanding and sense of agency within the relationship. Other caring attributes were noted, and these provide a model of caring to work with in this context. This way of caring captures first, the unique skills required to care for someone with DSI, and second, the self-care required for family carers to meet the demands of their caring role while maintaining their own identity within the caring dyad.

The art of caring in a DSI context includes empathic understanding; engagement in social networks; enabling a safe space, and social facilitation and protection; it also represents a bridging link between the caring dyad and broader social networks that may facilitate or limit social engagement, and which are recognized as crucial in maintaining social engagement (for both). Improving the art of caring in this context has the capacity to increase access to healthcare, enrich quality of care, and better understand the specific social and functional needs for those with DSI. Adopting this model of care may have benefits in improved health and well-being, a reduction of social isolation for the caring dyad, and economic savings.

Empathic understanding

Family carers play a critical role in creating and maintaining social engagement for their family member with DSI through understanding of DSI needs. This suggests that support and education for family carers may enhance reciprocal understanding and empathy. The availability of external support and level of awareness of DSI and its complexities, mediates empathy. One family carer described how empathy guided her actions; she noted how social encounters highlighted the invisibility of DSI to others, and shaped her understanding of when to intervene, particularly during negative social interactions:

> ……can hold his own, it's just that sometimes in a group situation people tend to have a conversation… you know they have eye contact, and they don't use names, you actually just have eye contact. So, if I'm speaking to you…I don't necessarily have to use your name, because you know I'm speaking to you. But [my husband] doesn't, he sits there, and someone's tried to say something to him and then when they don't get a response they turn away.
>
> (Family carer)

Social engagement

Family carers described the effort taken to encourage social participation with their family members, and the lengths they took to do this. Encouragement to "have a conversation, go to the local shops to pick a pint of milk up, go around instead of ringing her neighbor to ask something" (Family carer) was often met by reluctance from their partner or parent with DSI. Further communication support tactics such as "slowing… speech down…try and speak in the lower ranges so it's clearer, but [pretty much] I repeat everything" (Family carer) were used to encourage conversation. Despite these efforts, there was broad recognition of the gradual loss of cognitive processing ability and the motivation to encourage interaction was very often driven by these concerns of cognitive decline and potentially losing the art of conversation, integral to everyday social interactions.

Social facilitation and protection; enabling and destigmatizing

Understanding the social constructs of DSI created responsibilities for family carers to create and manage a safe environment. Safety involved both physical and social concerns. This also involved the facilitation of social interactions and networks to increase DSI visibility and destigmatize it for others. There is an art to balancing individual need for support with overprotection, and of encouragement versus forcing; these internal negotiations for family carers existed across all social networks, including during healthcare interactions.

The art of caring for self

Family carers experienced significant challenges in maintaining their social independence and identity. These challenges included, for instance, shrinking social networks and barriers to their own social participation, leaving little time to adapt to their ongoing changed circumstances as a family carer.

Family carers tended to adopt different ways of transitioning to the carer role, which could be either active or passive. Active and passive transitions represented a balancing act, with descriptions of this process suggesting elements of both co-existed. Active transition described intuitive and often deliberate ways of caring, while passive transitions were often arbitrary and incomplete. Early research (Dunsmore, 2022) suggests that the strength of carers' networks was potentially more important than gender in managing this transition effectively, although this needs further exploration and may differ with age.

Family carers range in age, health conditions, and other life and work commitments. While younger family carers generally experienced better health, they were also busy with other life commitments. In this context, strategies tended to be more practical, designed (often unintentionally) to help them adjust to their carer role. Younger family carers were often more intuitive than others to their own response to the more frustrating aspects of caring, recognizing their own needs as important: "it's two people to look after, not one" (Family carer). However, role ambiguity was pervasive: "I'm the carer, you know more than the daughter" and required skill and insight to manage effectively.

> I really have to think sometimes 'don't be frustrated about it.' Because it doesn't make any difference. The only person that suffers from that is me.

(Family carer)

Family carers often sought external support and demonstrated insight into the intangible social and communication aspects of DSI and the complex role they as carers, performed; however, family carers also recognized that maintaining their own identity within a caregiving relationship was an important, but complex, part of living effectively with DSI. As noted earlier, caring roles can be interchangeable in older adults and both may experience chronic illness or disability associated with age.

Active and passive transitions to a caring role

Family carers' transitioned to caring roles in different ways; some carers actively established their role, their support networks, and personal boundaries, which had social benefits for the dyad. Others had less flexibility in accessing external networks which impacted their resourcefulness in prioritizing their own needs. Considerations, such as an established and long-standing partnership with shared networks and familial obligations often meant shrinking networks and complex health needs (of their own). Difficulties might arise during this period of adaptation, often compounded by poor interpersonal communication and limited acknowledgment of the caring role. And of course, poor or limited external support intensified isolation for both.

Negotiating and maintaining social networks

Some family carers actively facilitated access to shared networks, often to the exclusion of their own. Maintaining independent networks, while important, was difficult; in the absence of strong family support, family carers looked to other external networks to help them in their caring role (see Chapter 6). While not specific to DSI, these external networks provided some opportunity for carers to engage in other social relationships (such as friends, social groups) separate to their relationship, that met *their* self-care needs.

Self-care is a critical component of caring and can support an easier transition to a caring role. While family carers experience caring differently, successful transition was embedded in the availability of appropriate social network support, which created shared opportunities and minimized their social isolation. The synergistic relationship of both elements of DSI caring—caring for others and caring for self—is an important aspect in the transition to a caring role.

The way forward: Caring in a DSI context.

Providing a way forward for those with DSI means that carers are central to both creating social opportunities and reducing social effort for their family member with DSI, enabling them to participate meaningfully. In summary, a caring model should include insight into the unique skills required to care for someone with DSI, and the self-care required for family carers to meet the demands of their caring role while maintaining their own identity within the caring dyad. This model of caring has four key attributes:

- Social facilitation and protection;
- Empathetic understanding;
- Engagement in social networks; and
- Enabling a safe space.

Caring in this way represents the bridging link between these microsocial features of caring within the dyad and the broader social networks that serve to both limit and facilitate social engagement in a DSI context.

1. Social facilitation and protection:
  - Bridging the conversation gap: Family carers play a crucial role in facilitating social interaction for their family member with DSI, and this appears dependent on the carer's level of empathic understanding of DSI and their sense of agency within the relationship. Family carers were responsible for understanding and interpreting social nuances, and it is clear that social rejection is often a shared experience. To avoid potential social disengagement for both, it is beneficial to engage in social events where support is available, to provide respite for the person with DSI and their family carer;
  - Redirecting the conversation, developing personal touch communication skills to facilitate social engagement; and
  - Acting as eyes and ears and providing social protection.

2. **Empathic understanding:**
   - Education and external support will facilitate empathic understanding. Education, in particular, needs to be focused on the dyad and centered around their individual and joint needs;
   - Empathy is modified by the presence of external support so there is an increasing need to provide targeted and DSI specific support that is person centered and inclusive of the family carer; and
   - Social responses need to be adapted to suit the social occasion. Many social encounters are difficult for those with DSI, so having a skilled communication partner and/or family carer is critical to facilitating conversation. Development of social haptics to facilitate communication is key to reducing interpersonal tension.

3. **Engagement in social networks:**
   - Engagement with social networks: understanding need and considering social effort and fatigue for both;
   - Accompaniment to support partner/parent in social circumstances; and
   - Encouragement to socialize, while also recognizing individual need.

4. **Enabling a safe space:**
   - Understanding the social constructs of DSI creates responsibilities for family carers to create and manage a safe environment;
   - Safety involves physical, social, and psychological concerns, which can add complexity to carer burden. This creates a need for broader social network involvement to support family carers in their role. Integration

of formal and informal carer networks is key to safe spaces; and

- Safety involves a whole of community approach and includes the facilitation of social interactions and networks to increase DSI visibility and destigmatize it for others.

Building social caring capacity in DSI–doing it better

In the absence of social support, family carers rely on other external networks to help them in their caring role. There is an absence of DSI support groups for those aging into DSI, meaning that, while not ideal, other support networks, such as low vision support groups, might provide some opportunity for carers to meet others in a similar situation. There is a clear need to adapt social caring roles to a DSI context and better integrate formal and informal carer networks that provide stability, skill, and recognition of the complexities of DSI. This means recognition as a unique and distinct disability and the building of dedicated support structures (see Chapter 6). We have highlighted key strategies and solutions for the family carer here and will discuss further in Chapters 7–10.

Conclusion

This chapter describes the role of family carers in a DSI context. Research narratives from family carers provide clear descriptions of the effort and art of caring in this context and, as such, provide some evidence-based strategies and recommendations which we detail in the above section "The way forward". To conclude, this section describes the social effort and social isolation involved in caring for a parent or spouse in the context of DSI and the challenges this poses to close relationships. Constant negotiations are required to effectively adapt to changing circumstances, often with no clear endpoint in the progression of their family member's DSI. The hidden and unrecognized social and physical consequences of DSI presented in previous chapters, shape the way carers are able to manage their caring responsibilities on a day-to-day basis. Their unique circumstances draw attention to the health *and* social issues of DSI, a central component of which is the intersectionality of DSI in these two domains that, in many ways, limits clear solutions. Family carers' insights offer an understanding of this at ground level; however, we also recognize the systemic barriers that shape the DSI experience and suggest that broader recognition, particularly at a primary care level, has the capacity to support carers and articulate clearer pathways to specific formal support for family carers in this context. Chapter 6 will focus on building social networks and how best to integrate formal and informal caring to provide support in a DSI context.

6

The impact of DSI on building and maintaining social networks

Introduction

This chapter reviews the social experiences of living with dual sensory impairment (DSI) and addresses the complexities of maintaining social networks in a DSI context. The recent World Health Organization (WHO) focus on loneliness as a global priority provides further justification to examine the invisible epidemic of DSI in older people, and its association with social isolation and loneliness. We explore the role of social networks in building and maintaining social participation and the impact of DSI on interpersonal relationships. We explore some strategies to build social participation that are person and family centered, drawn from the experiences of family carers (see Chapter 5). To understand the challenges of building and maintaining social engagement in a DSI context, this chapter will discuss the role of ageism, stigma, and self-stigma inherent in the experiences of aging into DSI. We consider the impact of the normalization and minimization of DSI which limits recognition and understanding of the effort involved in maintaining social networks for those with DSI.

The effort required to maintain meaningful social engagement when aging into DSI is particularly challenging, as it is often on a background of other age-related health challenges. There is significant pressure on those with DSI to continue socializing with family and broader networks but the lack of visibility of DSI means the effort involved and the support required remain hidden to broader social networks. Social activities, once pleasurable, become arduous, not least because of the barriers to participation: physical barriers, such as changed living circumstances and loss of community, such as moving from an established community to be closer to family, as well as the loss of driving, common to those with DSI, limit capacity to socialize independently. Additionally, social and communication barriers exist, compounded by the socioemotional and mental health effects of DSI. These barriers impact social enjoyment and the independence of those with DSI and demonstrate that communication, social networks, and family support are integral to those aging into DSI.

DSI at the intersection of aging and disability

DSI sits at the intersection of aging and disability paradigms which has a significant impact on older adults' understanding of DSI, their expectation of service delivery, and their personal expectations of "successful aging". The conflation of aging with a disability, such as DSI, presents a complex picture for older adults with DSI and their immediate social networks. This is highlighted by: i) Misunderstanding of DSI (by those with DSI and their social networks, as well as broader health and social care professionals) and internal acceptance of DSI *as part of* the aging process; ii) Existing social patterns and attitudes, such as stigmatizing attitudes to disability and aging; and iii) The lack of representation of DSI in all structures of society. With a rapidly aging population, all of these converge to create an invisible epidemic of DSI.

Effects of stigma and self-stigma

First, it is important to acknowledge that stigma and discrimination are central to the DSI experience in older age (and indeed any age) (Southall et al., 2010; Tian et al., 2020). Research has consistently identified stigma associated with hearing, vision, and dual sensory losses (David et al., 2018; Fraser et al., 2019; Shakarchi et al., 2020; Wallhagen, 2009, 2018), however, the lack of representation of *older adults* with DSI, and the poor diagnostic clarity of DSI in policy or healthcare maintains the perception that DSI experiences of exclusion and status loss are related to aging.

Stigma and social isolation present barriers to social participation for those with DSI, and there is also evidence of self-stigmatization (negative self-perceptions about hearing and/or vision loss). This relationship of individual perceptions and others' attitudes is seen in other sensory loss studies. For example, Fraser et al. (2019) reviewed barriers to rehabilitation for older adults with low vision, identifying four key themes, two of which related to stigma: i) The response and attitudes from others; and ii) Participants' own responses during social interactions. These negative attitudes and poor public understanding of sensory losses help explain the social withdrawal and disconnection from relationships by those with single sensory losses and DSI. Qualitative reviews by both Hersh (2013) and Lejeune (2010) provide similar observations of ostracism and social exclusion among those with DSI. This understanding of stigma and discrimination in a DSI context helps us better understand some of the barriers to maintaining and developing social networks for those with DSI.

Importance of social networks in older age

Social networks are important as we age. There is now widespread recognition and evidence for the connection between healthy social relationships and emotional and physical health across the life span (Berkman et al., 2000; Berkman and Syme, 1979; Holt-Lunstad et al., 2017), as well as how loneliness negatively impacts health (Cacioppo and Cacioppo, 2014; Holt-Lunstad et al., 2010, 2015). Global organizations, such as the WHO and United Nations, consider social support networks to be a key social determinant of health (WHO, 2021b), and the United Nations Convention on the Rights of Persons with Disabilities (UNCRPD) protects the right of all persons to participate socially (United Nations, 2006). Recent reports from the WHO (2019a) on integrated care for older persons support action in managing loneliness and social participation as a way of improving quality of life and managing decline in older people. Additionally, as a response to the post-Covid era, many nations are now explicitly embedding strategies to manage social participation and loneliness into their health and social care policies, for instance, in the UK and Japan, there are now Ministers for Loneliness, with strategic plans such as "Emerging Together: the Tackling Loneliness Network Action Plan" (UK Government, 2021) identifying systemic, organizational, community, and individual strategies to manage loneliness.

Loneliness and DSI

Social isolation (being alone or having infrequent social connections) and loneliness (the subjective and often upsetting feelings that originate from a mismatch between one's desired and one's actual social connection) often co-occur (Holt-Lundstad and Perissinotto, 2023). Older adults, in general, experience many age-related chronic health issues, poorer mobility, and decreased cognition, multiplying the potential for social isolation and loneliness. Older people with DSI very often have reduced social participation and smaller social networks (Mick et al., 2018) meaning that access to broader social support, education, and health information etc. can be limited. More broadly, sensory losses, including DSI, are associated with reduced social support and loneliness in older adults (Wang et al., 2022) through complex pathways underpinned by invisibility, stigma, and discrimination.

In Chapter 1, we observed the often tense social and healthcare interactions experienced by older persons with DSI. Without social support, navigating systems and organizations, healthcare or other, is complex and frustrating for those with DSI, impacting autonomy and capacity for shared decision making.

At a micro social level, lived experience studies provide detail of the significant effort involved in communication and social engagement:

> He doesn't talk anymore much, because he doesn't know whether they're talking to him, unless they use his name, he's unaware they're speaking to him, so he might ignore people and so on. And in the end, I noticed

> people weren't even bothering him to talk, so now I refuse to go. Because I don't think it's fair to Clive.
>
> (Carer)

This effort is in part responsible for the disengagement and reduced social participation seen in those aging into DSI. As noted in previous chapters, DSI limits speech perception and the ability to "join the conversation" at an appropriate point, leading to social embarrassment and gradual social disengagement despite the efforts of family carers, if present (see Chapter 5). Additionally, the effects of stigma and self-stigma, noted previously, limit help-seeking behavior and the provision of suitable support, if indeed available. Furthermore, those who accompany persons with DSI to their social engagements (such as family carers, family members, and friends) are often the first to recognize stigma and vulnerability, and therefore assume greater responsibilities to facilitate social engagement, protect and support their family member or friend during these encounters:

> He is not stupid, he's deaf. He's not stupid and I have become terribly protective of him you know. Particularly when he was in hospital, very protective of him, probably more so than I should have been.
>
> (Carer)

Social impact of DSI in older age

What do older persons mean by social support, social networks, and social participation? As you might expect, complex variations in support, networks, and participation exist across the lifespan, and are influenced by social circumstances, such as geography, and physical and mental health. Social networks (defined as the structural web of social relationships) are considered protective to health and well-being at all ages (Cornwell and Schafer, 2016). Social networks vary, for example, Granovetter's (1973) "weak" and "strong" ties suggest the *diversity* of networks and the presence of "weak ties" (i.e., more distant and diverse connections) remain important throughout life; others, such as, Antonucci (Convoy Model) suggest that social support is provided by a dynamic but ever-decreasing network of family and friends, who share life experiences and offer *reciprocal* support (Antonucci, 2001; Antonucci et al., 2014; Kahn & Antonucci, 1980). Although social networks are generally associated with improved access to social support (Holt-Lunstad, 2017), these networks can be limited in older age, or may fail to offer the *desired* social support (Bowling, 1991). We know that as network size decreases, older individuals focus on close relationships, which are central to support and adjustment (Cloutier-Fisher et al., 2011; Stephens et al., 2011). But what of older persons with DSI?

Smaller social networks and a reduction in network diversity may limit the provision of support, and access to information and resources, and perpetuate a cycle of missed opportunities for older adults with DSI (Jaiswal et al., 2020). On a superficial level, network reduction alone may provide some explanation for social isolation in DSI. However, the smaller, more microsocial changes associated with DSI, such as stigmatization, invisibility of DSI, and the increased interpersonal tension socially are key considerations too. It is also worth noting that for many older people (with and without DSI) larger social networks and new social groups are not necessarily the aim, rather, it is opportunities to have better social quality and communication with their established social networks that may improve quality of life.

Social networks and interpersonal relationships: Personal and interpersonal tension, connection, and disconnection

Micro social changes impact relationships, particularly close family relationships, such as the family carer: care receiver dyad. Literature from a range of health disciplines suggests wide acceptance of the interrelated health effects of illness and disability on both the impaired individual *and* their partner/caregiver (Antonelli et al., 2020; Braun et al., 2009). The interdependence and influence exerted within the family structure shape responses to stress (Randall and Bodenmann, 2009; Yorgason et al., 2006), their capacity to adjust to diagnosis, and psychological well-being for family members (Berg and Upchurch, 2007). These pathways have been used to explain relational stress in a number of diverse health domains such as cancer (Badr et al., 2010), chronic pain, and neurodegenerative disease such as dementia (Gellert et al., 2018). Bertschi et al. (2021) describes this as "we-stress" and highlights the potentially stressful impact of any chronic and disabling disease on the family unit and immediate social networks.

These changes can cause strain in close relationships and communication and can play a key role in older couples' ability to accept, adjust, and cope with relationship changes caused by ill health or disability (Horowitz et al., 2004). Recent qualitative research (Dunsmore et al., 2020) has explored what this means for the shared experiences and specific care needs of close family/family carers in a DSI context.

Close social networks and family carers play a role in helping their family member stay in a conversation, identify who is speaking, and find opportunities to engage in the conversation. This involves significant effort and can impact engagement and enjoyment of social occasions for others. "We-stress" (or relational stress) is observed in DSI, with impacted older adults and their close family members identified as being at risk of communication disruption (Barker et al., 2017; Heine and Browning, 2002; psychological distress (Kiely et al., 2020), and mental health issues (Lehane, Hofsöe et al., 2018). We-stress implies that the negative interdependent consequences of sensory loss, such as communication frustration, social isolation, and depression, may be predictive of similar effects in the non-impaired spouse (Bertschi et al., 2021; Lehane, Hofsöe et al., 2018). In this context, the resources required for coping may be limited or absent, given that, while partners and family members are critical to buffering the negative effects of sensory loss, they may have reduced capacity to do so. For family carers, particularly those who share their social networks with their family member with DSI, maintaining both their relationship *and* their social network is arduous:

> You have to basically modify your whole way of communicating, it's like being in a foreign country and you have to kind of more or less think that the other person is (you know), not able to understand you…so it's a constant strain
>
> (Carer)

Despite these inherent tensions, the limited data available on carer(s) and social networks in a DSI context suggest that family carers are critical to "bridging the social gap" and linking to broader social networks for their family member with DSI.

Integrating health and social support networks

As previously noted in Chapters 3–5, healthcare access and interactions, whether in hospital or primary care, are complex and often frustrating. Interactions with primary care and the healthcare system increase in frequency with age, with many older adults experiencing more than one chronic health condition (in addition to their DSI) which requires regular and longer interactions with healthcare professionals. Healthcare interactions are often characterized by poor communication, misinterpreted information, and loss of agency for those with DSI; this means that social support and protection are critical in this context. While these multiple health issues often take precedence over DSI, it should be noted too, that single and DSI also impacts morbidity and mortality, for example, cognitive decline and early mortality. Emerging research suggests that remediation of hearing loss has the capacity to reduce these risks.

General practitioners (GP) play a significant role in Australia in referring patients to specialist and allied health services, as well as managing and creating chronic disease plans. GPs are considered the first point of contact for the healthcare system. Both national and international research highlight the lack of DSI visibility in health professional knowledge, such that GPs had low recognition of the existence and complexities of DSI and often prioritize "other" health issues over DSI. Importantly, and in keeping more broadly with the poor recognition of DSI, the GP's professional response is more likely to fragment the two senses and refer for separate medical treatment, missing key opportunities to link participants to health and social support services and holistic rehabilitation services, such as Vision Australia, the specialist national organization, which has some capacity to address the complex needs of DSI, despite being a center for vision. This situation again highlights the need for distinct disability recognition for DSI, and government-funded dedicated DSI services.

This lack of access makes the role of social networks particularly important. Barriers to healthcare can occur at multiple levels: access to services in Australia is mainly through a GP, who act as a gatekeeper to all other services; those with DSI have reduced capacity to process information in a time-constrained consultation, and services are often physically and/or financially inaccessible. For the family and friends of persons with DSI, communication and agency are key concerns with healthcare professionals. Social networks, particularly close family, family carers, and friends, are critical to translating health messages, necessitating accompaniment to all health encounters to avoid key information being missed or misinterpreted. These health encounters are most often constrained by time, meaning little time to process information or seek clarification: "she's very nice, but she's in a big hurry" (older person with DSI). Qualitative research describes both family members and older adults with DSI as missing important information but feeling too embarrassed to request clarification: "some of these doctors forget us people" (older person with DSI), and a sense that they did not "understand fully what it's [DSI's] like" (older person with DSI). It is well established in the literature that poor communication is strongly associated with adverse events in healthcare and hospital settings (see Chapter 3).

Three-way communication between healthcare professionals, family carers, and those with DSI can be fraught. Inclusion is particularly important but often absent, making those with DSI feel excluded and disempowered, and creating a complex situation for family carers and friends. This is particularly so in situations where those with DSI feel unable to participate in health-related conversations or feel they are being talked about. In one narrative interview, a participant with DSI, recalled a recent encounter at hospital with one of her daughters:

> The surgeon came in and he was standing in front of [daughter] and myself, and I thought he was looking at me. It was [daughter] though, he was talking to her, and that's where I just stopped talking because it was pointless
>
> (older person with DSI)

Access to healthcare presented both physical and social challenges for participants. Those with DSI needed a family carer, or a family member to accompany them to health appointments, not simply to navigate the environment but also, to act as a default interpreter during consultations. Loss of privacy and poor communication strategies during healthcare interactions can impact older adults with DSI, and their accompanying friend or family member, with a reluctance to engage in healthcare conversations and subsequent disempowerment, often for both. It is critical to stress here that the legal and ethical responsibility for effective communication with patients with DSI, lies with the healthcare professionals (Hersh, 2013; Watharow, 2023).

Navigating social support

So, how do the close social networks of those with DSI, such as family and friends, manage this particularly complex mine-field: how do they navigate healthcare systems that disempower; how do family carers find support to understand and manage the complexity of DSI? The truth is—there is no rule book or cookie cutter solutions—many family carers (see Dunsmore et al., 2020; Kiely et al., 2020) develop *their own* strategies and build their own networks, in the absence of recognized external caring support.

This broader lack of role recognition mean that carers' efforts are relatively invisible to others in their broader social networks. As previously described in Dunsmore et al. (2020), family carers often lack critical understanding of, for instance, their social caring role: key roles such as social facilitation and being the "eyes and ears" for their family member are not necessarily aligned with their understanding or expectation of what caring means in this context. There was an understanding of the safety and physical aspects of their role, however, navigating the communication and social needs of those with DSI can be exhausting and relentless, limiting opportunities for independence for carers themselves, and potentially minimizing access to other potential webs of social support relevant to them as carers. The lack of recognition of their caring role by their family member with DSI, and others, added to the significant caring burden: "what can I say–they hardly seem to kind of recognize your own existence" (Carer).

In addition, those with DSI are very often reluctant to engage in other carer (formal or other) support, meaning carers lack space and time to process what is going on, to understand the nature of their caring role, and to plan ahead. Several factors can limit this: poor understanding of the variations in complexity and impacts of DSI, lack of GP and expert support for them as carers, and their own capacity (on a background of aging and co-morbidities of their own) to navigate changed circumstances and adopt new roles and identities. Potential solutions lie in supporting family carers to develop personalized strategies to support their family member as well as integrating care networks (both formal and informal) to provide a wider web of support for those with DSI. Additionally, some technologies are more suited than other more conventional technologies (such as mobile phone) with lived experience of some clients with DSI using a simple walkie-talkie (with a range of 3 kilometers) in an aged care facility. This was based on the fact that this married couple in aged care did not share a room and this device enhanced their feelings of safety; if she fell, it was her husband she contacted, not the nurses' station.

Building social network capacity

Building social network capacity is geared toward bridging a link between family social structures, community, and organizational structures that: i) Foster a safe space; ii) Facilitate positive social interactions; and iii) Create opportunities for independence for family, family carers, and those with DSI.

Systems and organizations play an important role in building social engagement in a DSI context. While other disabilities may provide support groups and external networks, this is not always the case for older adults with DSI. At best, support groups, such as vision impaired community groups local to Sydney, while not specific to DSI, provide an opportunity for family and friends accompanying their partner or parent with DSI to meet others in a similar situation. These support groups may provide incidental social opportunities and limited time out for family carers and family members, while not necessarily conferring the same benefits to the person with DSI.

Family carers can potentially play a crucial role in developing and maintaining important social networks to create safe spaces and facilitate social interaction for their family member with DSI. Significant effort is required and, at least in part, is dependent on the carers' level of understanding of DSI. Understanding is mediated by the availability of external health and social support, such as more formal (paid) carer support, assistance at home with activities of daily living (ADL), and the option of respite for carers. Formal (government-funded) service models of care generally provide intermittent task-orientated care, such as cleaning or personal care, rather than person-centered care: person-centered care means treating healthcare clients or patients as individuals and as equal partners in care; it is personalized, coordinated, and enabling. Person-centered care requires recognizing individual capabilities, and social and cultural context, and acknowledges clients as experts in their own health (Coulter and Oldham, 2016; McCormack and McCance, 2021). Task-orientated care underestimates the specific challenges faced by those with DSI. This may mean that communication difficulties are not considered central to care needs and suggests that family carers may find it easier to manage alone, rather than attempt to access non-specific resources that may not fulfill the social role required. While access to and recognition of the need for specific support is difficult, this may also occur in parallel to a reluctance by those with DSI to "share" care with anyone outside of family.

Building social networks and integrating caring capacity in DSI—doing it better

Current aged care support in the community (for example, home care packages; Commonwealth Home Support Program) provide support with activities of daily living but often neglect the more social aspects of caring required in a DSI context. Poor recognition and awareness of DSI, as well as a lack of training and support for the caring workforce, means that even when support is available it may not be fit for purpose. The Australian Government Department of Health runs the Commonwealth Home Support Program for aged care, which provides support for older adults over the age of 65 years, to remain at home independently with incremental levels of support (Australian Government, n.d.). For those under 65 years with DSI, there is the National Disability Insurance Scheme which has significant differences in level of provision and support from that of aged care, for instance, aged care packages for severe impairments may only provide a few hours of support, while the National Disability Insurance Scheme (for which you must be eligible prior to 65 years of age), provides significantly more for a younger person with DSI.

Different types of care exist relevant to need (Australian Government, 2020). These support packages may mean an opportunity for those with DSI to remain at home longer, with the support of family care. Sourcing appropriate and specific formal support is complex, with government-funded service provision for care of older persons in the community acknowledged as low-paid and insecure, with little specific communication training for supporting those with DSI. Those with DSI, and their family carers, report communication difficulties with these carers and the lack of choice and consistency in carer provision from the aged care package, means that families are reluctant to engage in this form of external care.

The provision of services does not often align formal carers with care recipient needs, making the development of carer relationships difficult. Additionally, formal care in a DSI context needs to support and understand the communication barriers experienced and foster family carer: formal carer relationship to provide integrated support. The provision of external support has the potential to reduce communication strain and potentially reduce interpersonal tension between family carers and those with DSI but requires careful planning, purposeful selection, and the opportunity to develop sustainable relationships.

In the absence of social support, family carers rely on other external networks to help them in their caring role. There is a clear need to adapt social caring roles to a DSI context and better integrate formal and informal carer networks that provide stability, skill, and recognition of the complexities of DSI. The recent World Federation for the Deafblind (2023) report identifies a number of key areas which we will focus on in Chapters 7–10. In terms of building social network capacity for older adults with DSI and their families, the WFDB (2023) report suggests the following:

1. Development of specific social centers, support groups, and resources to support older adults with DSI;

2. Services that are designed specifically for older adults with DSI;

3. Improving inclusion and accessibility, for example, in healthcare settings and in transport;

4. Education, training, and development of communication partners and formal/informal carers; and

5. Support for healthcare professionals to identify, rehabilitate, educate, and support older adults with DSI and their families.

However, it should also be noted that the development of these services, social centers, and DSI specific communication strategies requires co-design, and the inclusion of the DSI perspective at all levels, from design to implementation, noting the heterogeneity of DSI itself that means that no one size fits all. Additionally, the WFDB (2023) reiterates the need for DSI in older adults to be properly recognized in policy and legislative decisions, with the adoption of a definition that officially recognizes DSI as a distinct disability (p. 38).

We, as co-authors, acknowledge the lack of participation of older adults with DSI in the co-production of research, policies, and services in Australia, and as noted by the report (WFDB, 2023) and Simcock and Wittich, (2019). This book provides a starting point for the co-production of literature and the development of specific, tailored, and pragmatic strategies in the DSI context.

Conclusion

DSI is a complex condition associated with a number of communication, psychosocial, and functional impacts that shape capacity and desire to socially engage. The importance of social networks in aging is substantiated by research, and social networks both at a macro and micro level are integral to the support networks required for those with DSI. There is a pressing need to develop strategies that integrate formal and informal caring with organizational and system support. To do this, better policy recognition, professional education, and specific supports that highlight the social context of DSI and the complex interplay between the individual, their social networks, and the structural factors that limit participation in society, are required. Addressing the complex health *and* social issues of DSI, a central component of which is the intersectionality of DSI in these two domains, requires careful consideration, planning and development to structure a web of support that is skilled in managing the unique challenges of DSI. The following chapters, Chapters 7–10, adopt a pragmatic lens to address these challenges and support those with DSI to live better.

7
Living better

Communication 1: Basics for health and social care professionals/practitioners

Introduction

There is unfortunately a tendency for vision and hearing losses to be highlighted as individual and separate issues. Single sensory losses are better recognized in policy and research in Australia; dual sensory impairment (DSI) is less well known as a result of the lack of a distinct disability status. There are two significant reports (WHO, 2019b, 2021c) which identify global burden and the challenges associated with vision loss and hearing loss separately, but much less attention is attributed to vision and hearing loss in combination, as DSI. A recent World Federation of the Deafblind report (2018) points out that those with DSI are at risk of being excluded and further marginalized because of this lack of recognition. Countries with recognition of DSI as a distinct disability, such as the UK, provide legal recognition that enshrines: 1. Social care provisions; 2. Legal affirmation of the rights to accessibility and support; and 3. Credentialling of formal carers and support workers. In contrast, Australia's segregated treatment and service delivery limits understanding and means that attention to the complexities of communication is low.

This lack of recognition permeates health and social care education, as well as professional practice and policies. There are undeniable benefits to effective communication in relationships (reduced interpersonal tension and fewer misunderstandings, for example) and in health (better healthcare experiences and improved compliance with treatment plans, for example). This means that often communication awareness is lacking, which is where this book addresses an important gap. We believe an integrated and person-centered approach that takes account of the residuals of both senses, the resources of the individual and family, and the hopes, needs, and expectations of each older person living with DSI.

Here, we look at the simple strategies for improving communication. This section is designed to be indicative not exhaustive of the supports available to older people with single and dual sensory impairment. While people with sensory loss/es collectively may have difficulties in communication, accessing information, and navigating environments (orientation and mobility), these are experienced differently by each individual. So, every patient, client, member, and partner, must be asked what works for them, what doesn't, and what do they need. These responses need to be carefully considered and acted upon. We all need to be aware that communication needs are not always obvious, static, or the same.

Communication needs can change over time, and from day to day (e.g., from medication use, feeling tired, or anxious; variable use and effectiveness of hearing aids; sensory needs that may be undiagnosed). A lack of awareness of their sensory loss/es is common as many older people consider this as an unavoidable part of getting older. We cannot underscore enough the importance of being alert to the presence of sensory loss/es in patient and client encounters; and while some communication difficulties may be temporary, e.g., injuries, infections, and surgeries to ear/s and or eye/s, many are progressive.

With regard to accessibility technology (both low cost and more expensive), these are constantly changing fields. Accessibility features of smartphones, tablets, and laptops are frequently updated. This chapter will therefore not examine these exhaustively as up to the minute advice should be sought from hearing/vision rehabilitation services, support organizations, and accessibility technology consultants. It must be remembered that people living with DSI learn differently. Older people too have different capacities to manage little buttons, switches, and small font instructions. There may be technophobia. Many cannot afford the devices and training support as aged-care services usually don't provide funding for these. So, the resources available to each individual differ.

Wearing hearing aids is not a "fix it" for hearing loss. To dispel a common misconception, hearing aids do not restore hearing to "normal". Many wearers describe varied experiences that range from difficulties working the aids, pain or pressure areas from the moulds, difficulties in group settings with ambient noise amplified; others have positive experiences with improved one on one communication. Stigma (see Chapters 3 and 6) is more common with hearing aid use, and less common with wearing glasses.

Many who are prescribed aids refuse or discontinue wearing them, and this decision should be supported (see The House of Representatives (Commonwealth of Australia, 2017) "Still waiting to be heard…" report).

So, our message here is always ask and learn about the goals older people have, the difficulties they experience, what works and what doesn't. Then, work with the individual to see if the hearing aid can be reprogrammed to work better or another device trialed. This is especially important in light of emerging evidence regarding the role of hearing rehabilitation and reducing cognitive decline (e.g., Jiang 2023). Next, think creatively about solutions and hacks that might help. We begin here with simple strategies that family, friends, professionals, and support workers can incorporate to support the communication process. Then, we will mention in brief some low-cost accessibility technologies. We will also look explicitly at how professionals in health and social care can better support communication for important conversations. These strategies don't just apply to older people with known DSI. They apply to anyone and everyone who has any form of communication difficulty, whether temporary or permanent.

Author One's experience is that we don't do enough in social and health domains to support people living with DSI. We don't take the time to learn. We don't prioritize this as a distinct disability or as a focus in specific health policies and integrated care services, nor do we have space on curricula in health and social care courses. One research participant had this to say about their DSI experiences:

> One minute you can be in an environment that's nice and quiet and you're familiar with. The next minute a few

people enter the room, things get moved and people are talking and you've just lost control. You can't communicate any more. People tell me I am a confident person, a capable person. I am, you just have to put me in a room with three people and I go sight-hearing impaired shy. I turn shy because I can't hear what is going on, and I can't see what is going on, so I can't say anything. I can't participate.

(Dunsmore, 2022)

Simple strategies for everyone

- ASK what communication support is needed
- Face the person you are communicating with
- Speak clearly
- Speak at a moderate or slower pace
- Wear strong colored lipstick, e.g., red, to help in finding your mouth and watching what you are saying. This can really help lip-readers
- Remove masks where possible
- Ensure the lighting is optimal for the individual (some need bright lights; others may need dimmer lighting to counter contrast sensitivity)
- Move to a quieter location as ambient noise (if other conversations in the room, in a restaurant, or on a busy street for example may inhibit communication)

Basic dual sensory impairment communication supports

We will now look at specific basic communication strategies for older people with DSI.

How do you introduce yourself to a DSI person?

- Wave!
- Waving in the visual field (if visual field is restricted wave in the center, if central vision is reduced, e.g., in age related macular degeneration, wave away from the central vison)
- Speaking clearly
- Light touch in a safe area, e.g., hand, shoulder, arm
- Check where are the safe areas to touch on the body: usually hands, shoulder, and upper arms. But always ASK

Basic communication with a person with DSI

- Keep eye contact and face toward the person
- Close body language and gesture
- Point and use facial expression
- Speak clearly (No need to speak loudly or over-enunciate)
- Large font writing
- iPad/phone speech to text features, use white or yellow writing on black background if that helps improve contrast

Basic guiding to communicate environmental information

- Always stop/pause before any change in terrain, escalators, stairs, or curbs. Touch messaging is not always instantaneous, so stop. Also, pause before uneven ground and give a signal with your fingers moving around quickly and randomly to indicate the rough ground
- Normal walking

- o   Their hand on your elbow by your side or some prefer to place their hand on your shoulder
- Narrow areas
  - o   Your arm behind your back to signal a tight squeeze, e.g., between parked cars
- Stairs up
  - o   Lift your shoulder, pause then ascend slowly
- Stairs down
  - o   Drop your shoulder, pause then descend slowly
- Guide to a chair
  - o   Your hand under their hand, to back of chair and perhaps seat
- When it is safe to do so, give some visual description of the environment. Don't walk and talk at the same time unless the person with DSI has enough residuals to do so. Many need to concentrate on being safe
- Use the manual alphabet, short cuts messaging, and social haptics to supplement visual description if needed and used by the individual

Low-cost measures and accessibility technologies

Hearing loss

Hearing difficulties are very common in Australia with 66 percent over 60 experience hearing loss, a number that continues to increase as the population ages (The House of Representatives

(Commonwealth of Australia, 2017) "Still waiting to be heard…" report). Hearing loss is also more common for people with other disability or health conditions. Hearing loss is often overlooked in the presence of other impairments or misdiagnosed, e.g., as a cognitive impairment. As well as the basic communication supports outlined earlier, accessibility devices may be useful to improve communication and access to information.

Hearing impairment communication supports

- Using paper or whiteboard and marker to write down what you are saying
- Speech to text apps such as Otter AI
- Hearing aids
- Cochlear implants
- Personal amplifiers
- Headphones
- National Relay Service (Government service offers a variety of communication relay methods; chat, speak and read, type and read, etc.)
- Telephone amplifiers (built into the receiver of the telephone can help increase the volume for the listener. In addition, for those who have difficulty hearing the high-pitched ring of the telephone, the sound can be replaced with a lower tone bell or buzzer, or with a visual alert)
- Captioning and transcribing (captioning films and video meetings, and transcribing events, meetings, etc.)
- Roger Pen (a high-tech microphone which facilitates better hearing in complex sound environments)

- Loud doorbell chimes (some doorbells can be connected via Bluetooth to another device (such as a smartphone), to make the device vibrate when someone rings the bell)
- Vibrating smoke alarms connected to a smartphone or watch via Bluetooth, so the device vibrates when the alarm goes off
- Accessibility features on smartphones and tablets are evolving all the time and up to date advice should be sought from accessibility technology specialists

Low vision

Low vision is increasingly common as we age. There is a rapidly increasing prevalence of acquired visual impairment due both to population growth and aging, with the number of those with acquired vision loss expected to double in most Global North countries over the next three decades (Varma et al., 2016). The prevalence of low vision in Australia from 2021 is expected to double by 2050 (AIHW, 2020). Alongside basic communication measures as above those with low vison or blindness can benefit from a range of accessibility provisions.

Vision impairment communication supports

- National Relay Service (Government service offers a variety of communication relay methods; chat, speak and read, type and read, etc.)
- Describing the layout of the room using a clock analogy (i.e., describing the person with vision impairment as 12 o'clock and relating those in the room/things in the room to a clock face)

- Text to speech on smartphones, tablets, and laptops
- Smart canes–An electronic travel aid which fits over a white cane and enhances the cane's ability–detecting things above the knee (Rohan et al., 2007)
- Ultrasound devices, e.g., miniguide (these convey information about the environment through ultrasound and vibration)
- Braille reader device (requires someone to be transcribing)
- Screen reading technology, e.g., a free-to-the-user screen reader created by blind people in Australia for blind people called NonVisual Desktop Access NV Access; a commercial example is JAWS
- Braille labels and adhesive sheets to label household items such as cleaning solutions, canned goods, etc. (widely available from various online stores, also available from Vision Australia and is National Disability Insurance Scheme [NDIS] consumable eligible.
- Screen magnification (most devices have some capability to do this on their own, additional magnification software is widely available online)
- DAISY Devices (DAISY is an acronym standing for "Digital Accessible Information System". These digital reading systems help make audiobooks accessible to individuals with visual difficulties that affect their ability to read printed material)
- Accessibility features on smartphones and tablets are evolving all the time and up to date advice should be sought from accessibility technology specialists

Especially for health and social care professionals

Registered Nurse/GP/allied health professional/social worker/ support worker means that you need to:

- ASK what is needed for good communication, then act on it;
- SCREEN for sensory loss;
- SUPPORT patient/client and family with education, reassurance, referral strategies, and referrals;
- PROVIDE preventive care;
- DIAGNOSE co-occurring conditions early;
- ENSURE REGULAR CHECK-UPS as many conditions causing sensory loss are degenerative;
- ALLOW TIME to deal with communication and complexities;
- TAKE RESPONSIBILITY for good communication;
- BE A BETTER COMMUNICATOR by following these strategies and then checking that the information has been correctly received; and
- BE PART OF A "SUPER TEAM" for the older person with DSI, more on this shortly.

Super teams

One crucial way that health and social care professionals and practitioners can help older people with DSI (in fact any older persons) is to be a part of a super team providing care, support, and capacity building. We can help people with DSI and their families build a team of GPs, registered nurses, allied health professionals, specialists, social workers, psychologists, hearing rehabilitation, and orientation and mobility experts. Each team will be different as each person has different residuals of hearing and vision, different goals, and different personal resources. Don't forget to include the partners, families, and carers in the super team. Have meetings, share ideas, and educate each other. This is exceptionally important for all older people. See Melissa Levi's book "We need to talk about ageing" (Levi, 2023). This resource has clear advice on how to achieve a dream super team.

Better communication

It is our/your responsibility to ensure that effective communication for all important conversations happens. As noted in previous chapters, poor communication can lead to adverse health outcomes as patients have longer hospital stays, more frequent readmissions, increased presentations to emergency departments, lower health literacy and understanding of health information, and poorer patient experiences. These are all strongly associated with decreased health and well-being. In addition, patients may delay seeking further health support, compromising their future health and well-being. The onus for communication is on us, the health and social care professionals and practitioners, as a legal and ethical responsibility.

These are some helpful strategies to assist our patients, clients, and members to know what is going on:

- Do the research and learn about DSI and the different causal conditions;
- Be person centered: Read the medical records and understand what is known so far about the person with DSI;
- Recognize that not everyone has a visible disability: Persons with DSI may have no outward signs that they have a

communication issue, so be alert to this possibility in all patient and client encounters;

- ASK, always: This nice acronym refers to "Acquiring Specific Knowledge" (Watharow 2023) by asking the person with DSI: What works for them? What do they need? Responsibility to acquire knowledge and skills about the conditions and communication needs of our patients and clients, is ours, as health professionals and practitioners;

- Choose a good environment for communication: A noisy office or ward is not the place. Find somewhere quiet without glare. Don't have older people with DSI looking into windows as their cataracts make it hard to see well. Ask the patient/client if they need a brightly lit space or a dimmer one;

- Face the person and speak clearly, at a moderate pace;

- Take off your mask to enable lipreading if possible (Ministry of Health mandate in August 2020);

- Book interpreters if needed, e.g., Auslan or CALD;

- Provide accessible formats to all your forms, information, brochures etc. Large print also rules the world for people over 40 who have forgotten their reading glasses. Accessibility also applies to all the research you do and the evaluations you perform of your services. It is hard to provide feedback if the form is not accessible;

- Keep up to date: Accessibility technology is a constantly changing and evolving phenomenon. We won't go into great detail here because of this. It is incumbent on professionals working with people with sensory loss/es to stay up to date in this rapidly shifting area;

- Allow extra time to relay, check, and answer questions and for information to be absorbed. Research suggests for people with DSI, a double appointment may be needed (Moller and Deci, 2005);

- Pivot if one method isn't working. Don't be frustrated and don't shout. That just stresses everyone and also risks being abusive;

- Own your accent, know that many older people will be polite and just say yes to everything that is said, even when they have not understood or heard. So, acknowledge your accent may contribute to difficult communication, and use another method if speaking is not working;

- Be creative: Use speech to text; text to speech; pen and paper; whiteboards and pen; personal amplifiers with disposable covers; use flash cards;

- Learn from people with DSI, and their families. You don't need to be an expert in using all devices: You can ask clients and their family members for advice about how to use and support them using a device. Additionally, use the internet to find plain language instructions;

- Check: What has your patient, client, or member understood? How many milligrams of prednisone? 15? 50? Repeat information and revisit at the next consultation; and

- Recognize, certify, and advocate: Health and social care professionals can help older people with DSI by recognizing when sensory losses occur, and certify what is going on (the DSI), advocate for that individual (more at home support, devices etc.), and make the necessary referrals. Be responsive and efficient, help older people get what they need to kick goals and live happier, healthier, and safer lives.

Acquire skills and knowledge

This means positioning yourselves/ourselves as a learner. Embrace that we are all learning how to communicate better with each other. ASK (acquire skills and knowledge) to help better communicate with clients and patients as well as ASKING the person with DSI what they need. Help older people with DSI to embrace lifelong learning by learning new ways of doing things. This is critical if a transition to tactile messaging is needed.

Managing specific conditions

The first important management principle is to be aware of common conditions and the role sensory loss plays in their increased frequency.

We will look very briefly at some of these:

- Communication breakdown;
- Depression;
- Anxiety;
- Delirium;
- Visual hallucinations (see Chapter 4);
- Increased mortality;
- Cognitive decline;
- Falls;
- Health literacy impacts; and
- Poor hospital experiences.

As health and social care workers, we need to encourage those living with sensory loss, single and dual, to see their health professional regularly. This way chronic conditions can be managed effectively, encouraging early diagnosis of conditions predisposing to delirium, e.g., urinary tract infections (UTI), and increasing support if sensory loss worsens or an additional sensory loss develops. In addition, health professionals should ensure that they check the hearing and vision of all their older patients yearly so that losses are detected earlier. We will look briefly at some common conditions experienced by those living with sensory loss.

Communication breakdown

Communication breakdown is common (Heine and Browning, 2002, 2004) as we have established in this book. Strategies have been outlined in earlier and subsequent chapters.

Anxiety and depression

We challenge the myth that anxiety is a normal part of aging. Anxiety is common in all older people (around 10–15% according to Bryant et al., 2008) and more common in those with DSI (Simning et al., 2019). It is not inevitable nor is it untreatable. We challenge the myth of getting older that depression is a normal part of aging. It's common in all older people (around 10% (Pirkis et al., 2009), and very common in those with DSI (Simning, 2019)); it is not inevitable nor untreatable. More worryingly, 60 percent of residents in residential aged-care experience one or more mental health conditions (Amare et al., 2020). DSI is common in those living in care and is often undiagnosed and/or un/under supported (Pavey et al., 2009).

Levi, a clinical psychologist in an older age mental health service, in their book *We Must Talk About Ageing* writes, "Prior to working with older people, I held two false (and rather dangerous) beliefs. One was that becoming depressed, anxious, lonely, and withdrawn was an inevitable part of growing older. The second was there was nothing that could be done about it. One of the greatest lessons that I have learned over the past decade is this: depression and anxiety are not inevitable, normal parts of the aging process. I have also learned that happiness, joy, meaning, wonder, hope, vitality, growth, confidence and an immutable zest for life are natural and normal parts of getting older" (Levi, 2023). Clearly having a psychologist, older age mental health specialist, or counselor on a super team makes sense to support older people re-attain life.

Increased mortality risk

Researchers have noted an increased mortality risk (Gopinath et al., 2013; Lee et al., 2007; Zhang et al., 2020) for older people living with DSI. The pathway is complex, however, better diagnosis and support of sensory impairments in primary care will ensure that the risks we have described are minimalized for each individual. Living unsupported means that difficulty with activities of daily living and instrumental activities of daily living (Brennan et al., 2005; Brennan et al., 2006; Guthrie et al., 2018) will occur. Another reason why everyone involved in the care of an older person with DSI is part of a super team.

Cognitive decline

It is increasingly evident that single and dual sensory loss are associated with higher rates of cognitive decline (Davidson and Guthrie, 2019; Livingstone et al., 2020, Lin et al., 2004; Tay et al., 2006). It is important that super teams be alert to symptoms of cognitive decline and adjust their communication appropriately. Those with DSI need to be included in discussions around health and well-being, but more effective communication modes are needed in this scenario. The use of different communication modes, e.g., whiteboard and thick pens, drawings, speaking slowly, and repeating content each consulation and over time is crucial. Limit content to what is really important. Be patient.

Delirium

Older people with DSI are more likely to develop delirium (Cacchione et al., 2003). Delirium is a serious change in mental abilities, it results in confused thinking and a lack of awareness of one's surroundings (Inouye et al., 2014). Common causes are urinary tract and other infections, medication side effects such as opioids for pain relief/falls.

Management includes:

- Urgent clinical review;
- Maximize sensory function: This means diagnosing sensory loss promptly;
- Ensure all aids, including hearing aids and glasses, are in place to help with orientation. It is also important to make sure they work! Replace batteries regularly (Author One is in favor of battery Monday where batteries are replaced each week for those living in Residential Aged Care (RAC). Ensure tubing is intact and is not blocked with wax;
- Communicate clearly, slowly, and calmly with the patient, reorientating and reassuring as delirium IS a distressing experience; and

- It is beyond the scope here to address clinical management of delirium but obviously the underlying cause needs to be quickly addressed.

Falls

Falls are a common cause of morbidity and mortality in older people and more common for those with DSI. So, prevention of falls becomes an important part of navigating older age for those with DSI. Engage occupational therapists and low vision support agencies to help make homes safer for older people living with DSI. Ensure that support/carers doing sighted-guiding have training with the older person with DSI, and seek further formal training for the person with DSI. Confidence going forward in familiar and unfamiliar environments is an important skill to learn, and re-learn if there is further deterioration in impairments or the acquisition of new ones. Fall detectors may be useful to enable early assistance after an accident.

Visual hallucinations and Charles Bonnet syndrome

Visual hallucinations are very common in older people, and more common in older people with DSI (Pang, 2016; Vukicevic and Fitzmaurice, 2008). They can be experienced as part of dementia, Parkinson's disease, psychiatric disorders, and delirium.

The triad of vivid visual hallucinations, low vision, and intact cognition is usually benign and called Charles Bonnet syndrome. Charles Bonnet syndrome is very common, affecting one third of people with low vision (Jones et al., 2021) (see Chapter 4). Seeing the unseen is more common in older people and can be distressing and misdiagnosed. Those experiencing hallucinations benefit from early diagnosis with a good history, examination, and investigation. This should be followed by reassurance, information, and support. In a few cases, with persistent distressing visions, anti-anxiety, antidepressant, or antipsychotic medications may be required. Behavioral strategies are often helpful, such as rapid blinking, increasing lighting, playing music, going for a walk etc. See Chapter 4 for more detail.

Health literacy

It is not surprising that DSI can impact health literacy in negative ways. Reduced access to information and communication failures combine to compromise shared decision making in healthcare. Therefore, providing integrated care will ensure that older people with DSI understand their healthcare plan and future management. We need to be alert when we are having important conversations with our clients and patients. Health literacy varies depending on multiple factors, so specific strategies are needed to address this in face-to-face communication. In addition to the simple strategies listed above, there are the following:

1. **ASK** what works and learn what doesn't. Offer different supports/reasonable adjustments—sometimes people do not know they can ask for these. To do this you must have a good idea of what the spectrum of communication can look like, and what reasonable adjustments you can offer;

2. **BE AWARE** of diagnostic overshadowing. This means assuming a medical symptom is related to a person's disability rather than another health issue. It is important to try to understand what the person's baseline communication is like;

3. **ASSESS** baseline understanding: Find out what the person already knows on a topic;

4. **EXPLAIN**

   a. Avoid medical jargon
   b. Use the patient's words
   c. Use plain language
   d. Check for understanding (use teach-back). See free training at www.teach-back.org. Teach-back puts the onus on the clinician to make sure they've explained things clearly. The clinician asks the patient to explain the health advice in their own words so they can see if anything was not communicated clearly;

5. **REPEAT CONTENT**

   a. Prioritize what needs to be discussed
   b. Limit to 3–5 key points
   c. Repeat
   d. You may need to use multiple modes, e.g., oral explanation, large print written materials to take home;

6. **VISUAL SUPPORT MATERIALS** (after you have ascertained they have sufficient vision as many, e.g., with age related macular degeneration, have blurred central vision):

   a. Use pen and paper, images or models
   b. Demonstrate instructions
   c. Provide accessible to the patient materials to take home
   d. Links to web pages, video etc. are useful ONLY if you have ascertained they are accessible to this patient at this time;

7. **ENCOURAGE QUESTIONS** Asking "What questions do you have?" is more effective than asking "Do you have any questions?" or "Do you understand?" This lets patients (and their families) know you are expecting questions and have time to respond. This is important for older people with and without DSI as many don't want "to be a bother";

8. **CREATE A SAFE SPACE** This means ensuring conditions in the room are optimal for communication and is a place where older adults are empowered to ask questions and clarify what is being said. Reduicng ambient noise is critical. Mishearing drug doses is something we see in people with hearing loss where three, thirteen, and thirty sound similar, writing it down can avoid dangerous errors. The onus is on us as professionals and practitioners to get communication right, so check understanding and incorporate teach-back into your practice (teach-back resources are listed at the end of the chapter);

9. **TAKE HOME MATERIALS**

    a. Write down important instructions (after ascertaining that the patient has sufficient vision)

    b. Educational materials to take home. Ensure these are in accessible to the individual patient formats. Large print, extra-large print, or braille may be needed

    c. Make an audio recording on the patient's smartphone for them to listen to later if low vision or use text to speech/speech to text applications to provide what the patient needs; and

10. **ACCESSIBLE CONSENT FORMS**: Always, always provide an accessible to the patient consent form. We have a legal and ethical obligation to do this, but in practice it rarely happens.

Useful resources

Communication training modules

- Teach-back: Teachback.org
- Communication Hub, see for example Supporting Communication
- Scope Australia Communication Access
- Language Guide—People with Disability Australia (pwd.org. au)
- Learning Hub: Neurodiversity affirming practice
- Council for Intellectual Disability: Communication Tips
- NSW Clinical Excellence Commission:

  o Person-centered care—Clinical Excellence Commission (nsw.gov.au);
  o Safety Fundamentals for Person-Centered Communication—Implementation Guide (nsw.gov.au)

Patient self-advocacy

- **Top 5** TOP 5 Initiative (nsw.gov.au); TOP 5 Toolkit—Hospital (nsw.gov.au)
- **My Health Matters** My-Health-Matters-Folder-Council-for-Intellectual-Disability.pdf (cid.org.au)
- **All About Me** (Sydney Children's Hospital Network)
- **Sunflower Symbol** A symbol for non-visible disabilities, also known as hidden disabilities or invisible disabilities. (hdsunflower.com)
- **Julian's Key** www.health.qld.gov.au/public-health/groups/ disability

Written resources to support face-to-face communication

- Say Less Show More | Agency for Clinical Innovation (nsw. gov.au)

Conclusion

Good communication, education, and reassurance are important therapeutic tools that we can give people with DSI and their carers/families. Older age with DSI is not an inexorable, inevitable state of loneliness, depression, anxiety, falls, chronic illness, frailty, and decline. Building our super teams for people with DSI and their carers/families, means we can make a difference. Helping our clients and patients with DSI be prepared for health and hospital encounters will instill confidence and reassurance. Educating older people with sensory loss, their families, and carers on screening, support, and common co-occurring conditions will improve prevention and early detection.

8
Living better

Communication 2: Social-haptic communication

Introduction

People have been using on-body touch signals for centuries. Most people use tactile gestures to signify support (patting on the back) and love (holding hands, kissing) for example. People with a disability and their families have sometimes created idiosyncratic, informal, and individual systems when sighted-hearing-speaking senses are singly or multiply compromised or not available as a conduit for communication.

The formal counterpart to these informal messaging systems is social-haptic communication (Palmer and Lahtinen, 2013). Note, we are not talking about tactile languages such as hand-over-hand Australian sign language or Pro-tactile, American sign language. What we are talking about here is a quick messaging system that is both formal and can also allow innovation for individual and group needs.

Social-haptic communication

Social-haptic communication is a system of on-body tactile messaging; shortcuts as it were. It can take years to learn a language but days or weeks to learn a formal tactile system like social-haptic communication.

Definition

Social-haptic communication is "touch messages between two or more people in a social context (person-to-person)" (Palmer and Lahtinen, 2013, p. 68). This is different to haptic communication which refers to technology devices using vibrotactile elements to convey information, e.g., vibrating mobile phone, Buzz™ watch, computer, or gaming joystick. These can also have a role in supporting communication and access to information for those with single and dual sensory impairment, but this is not the subject of this chapter.

A communication arsenal

The social-haptic communication framework can be used to generate new symbols for different needs, hobbies, events, and situations. Social-haptic communication is best used as dictated by what the individual needs and wants, and what works well with other systems such as manual alphabets, tactile sign language/s, and other communication methods.

The ability of social-haptic communication to be part of a wider information system is of particular benefit to older people with dual sensory impairment (DSI), who will mostly have retained some hearing between and or some sight. Older people with acquired DSI have well established communication modes that served them well before the onset of sensory loss/es. After DSI, these are not working quite as well anymore as neither sense can compensate for the loss of the other. And there is usually some time that elapses before the impacts are felt. For many, there is a hermeneutic gap in their understanding of what is happening as communication competencies erode (Dunsmore, 2022). This is where social-haptic communication can help contextualize, fill gaps, and support social and healthcare encounters in simple, discreet, on-body messaging ways.

History of social-haptic communication

The systematization of social haptics began with a meeting over 30 years ago at a conference in Sweden between Russ Palmer, a music therapist with Usher syndrome (causing DSI), and Riitta Lahtinen, a communication specialist, working with deafblind and blind clients. A personal and professional co-creation process was set in motion.

Social-haptic communication is an evolving, living entity as the years from inception have resulted in the ongoing addition of new haptices (touch messages). One thing that makes the system we are describing here as the most relevant and useful, is the co-creation between a person with deafblindness and a practitioner of communication support and interpretation for those with sensory losses.

Lahtinen and Palmer began innovating, refining, and researching from 1993 onwards. Lahtinen formally systematized social haptics in her doctorate in 2008. Palmer explains that social-haptic communication methods are usually combined with linguistic information. This gives a greater in-depth quality of information to the deafblind user, while at the same time providing shortcut methods and real-time information flow (Palmer and Lahtinen, 2013).

Social-haptic communication has spread with translations, courses, publications, and educational modules in the UK, Europe, Nordic countries, and Russia (Palmer and Lahtinen, 2013).

In brief, social-haptic communication can:

1. Provide a framework for quick social, emergency, health, and environmental messaging;

2. Evolve with new haptices (touch messages) added and allow creation of individual haptices;

3. Allow emergency messaging and this is important in assisting emergency personnel to gain cooperation and for people who use social haptics to understand what is going on and what is needed;

4. Communicate body language to a person with DSI, e.g., nodding, smiling;

5. Enable real-time messaging, there is no or minimal relay delay;

6. Include name sign equivalent of "body name" to identify who is speaking, who is here, and who is leaving;

7. Use body mapping to convey environmental information, e.g., who is sitting where in a restaurant, the ground is uneven;

8. Be applied in a wide variety of situations: at home, with family and friends, in restaurants, meetings, hospital settings, out and about, travel etc.; and

9. Combine with spoken language, sign language, tactile languages, and manual alphabets.

(Lahtinen, 2008; Lahtinen and Palmer, 2005; Palmer and Lahtinen, 2013)

How to use social haptics
Establish safe touch zones

While touch messaging is generally conducted on the arm, shoulder, or hands, it is important to establish safe touch zones with the person being communicated with. Asking about safe touch areas is crucial for people with neurodivergence who may not wish to be touched at all, or only in one specific location. Haptics may not be suitable or comfortable for everyone and a pivot may be needed to another method.

It can be useful to use a cut out paper doll for people learning social-haptic communication and ask them to map out safe zones (and/or "no-go") zones.

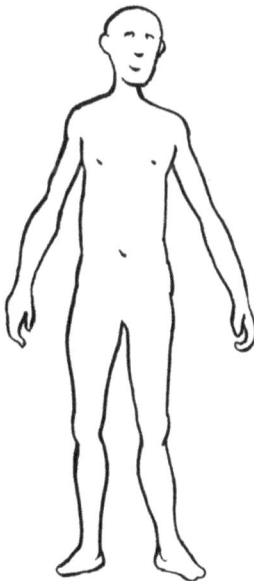

Image: an example of where safe zones may be mapped on the body

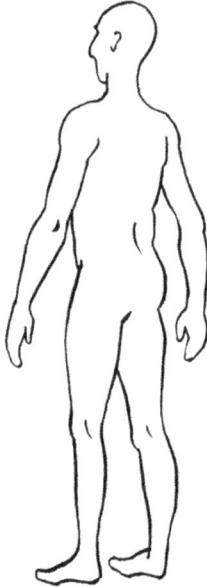

Haptices and Haptemes

Social-haptic communication is made up of haptices and haptemes. **Haptices** (touch messages) are the words, which are combined with haptemes, also known as grammar elements. Examples of grammar elements include the pressure of the touch such as soft/light, firm/heavy, speed (fast or slow), the type of movement (tapping, up/down/circular/random or patterned), and hand shape (such as fist or flat hand). The location of the touch may also be a hapteme (grammar element), e.g., shoulder or hand.

Examples

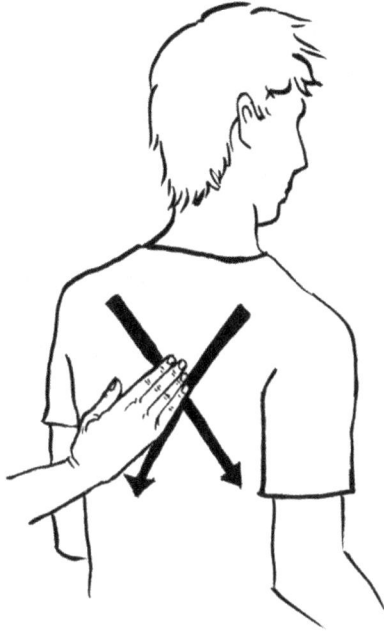

a.   Emergency

This is the most important haptice and should be taught to all people with a communication disability. Draw a large "X" on the person's back using the palm or blade of the hand or finger. This means: There is an emergency come with me immediately and I will explain later. Lahtinen and Palmer note that this is an International haptice. Author One has taught the building supervisor and security where she works to use the emergency haptice. This means if she is working alone and there is an emergency or evacuation order, staff can communicate this in real time and she will follow.

b.   Yes/no

These were the first developed haptices in 1994, and mimic the movement up and down of the head for YES and the sideways shaking of the head for NO.

Yes: Closed fist moving in a nodding motion up and down

OR

Finger moving up and down the arm, or up and down on the palm of the hand.

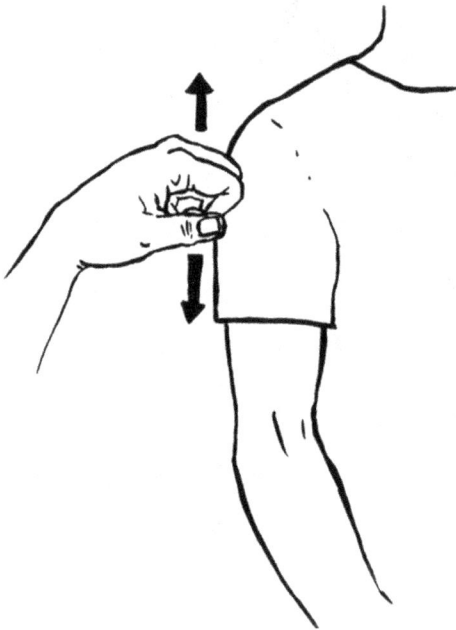

No: Closed fist moving in a shaking motion left-right-left-right

OR

Fingers doing a rubbing out motion on the upper arm or the palm of the hand.

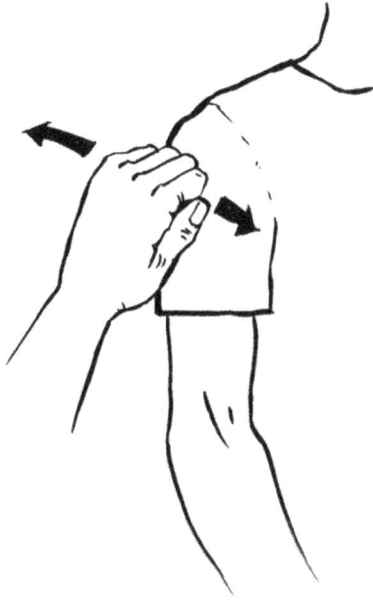

Maybe: Closed fist with only thumb and little finger extended. This can be done in space, on a shoulder, arm, or hand.

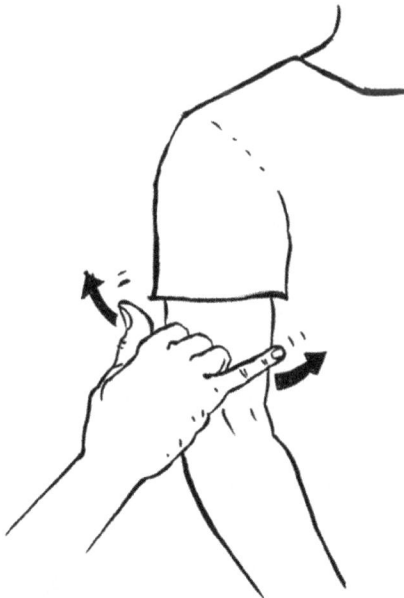

Environmental description

Environmental description of what is around the person with DSI can be conveyed by body mapping.

A room, café, restaurant, meeting room, lounge or sitting room, dining table etc. Starting at the center of the upper back with two hands trace the shape of the room.

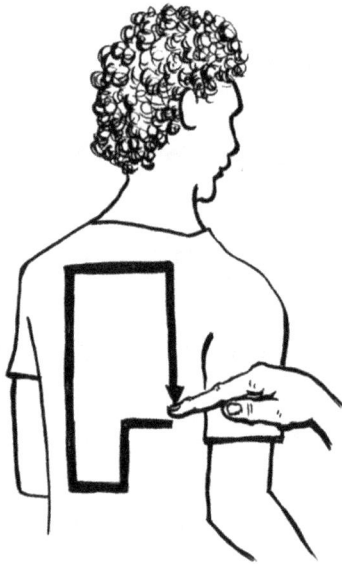

Next, it is important to place the person receiving social-haptic communication in the mapped-out space. This helps the person to work out where other objects such as doors, tables, or chairs are for example, and also where other people are situated in the space relative to where they are standing or sitting. After mapping the outline of the space, place the person in the map.

In a restaurant or around a meeting table, you would map the shape of the room and then the dining table. Use the index finger or first finger and second finger side by side, to indicate where the person with DSI is sitting. Others around the table can then be orientated using the index finger to point their location around the table. You might speak, use a manual alphabet, or a name sign/body name to indicate who is where. In this way mapping/drawing out the room and the locations of contents and people allows the person with DSI to mentally visualize their surroundings. For some with a loss of central vision, for example, due to age-related macular degeneration, they may not be able to see faces and objects directly in front. Mapping in this way improves social confidence (and safety). Exits can also be mapped on the back as well.

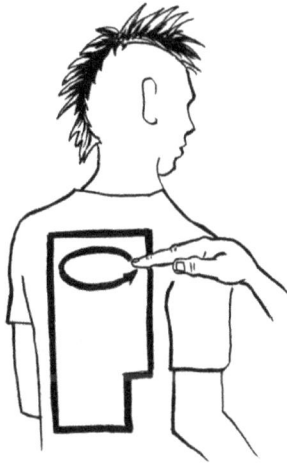

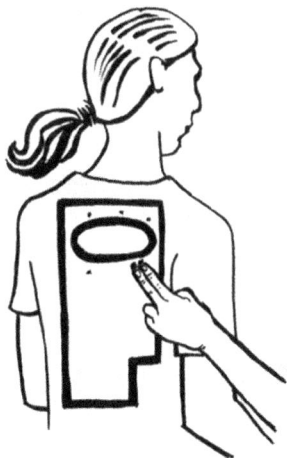

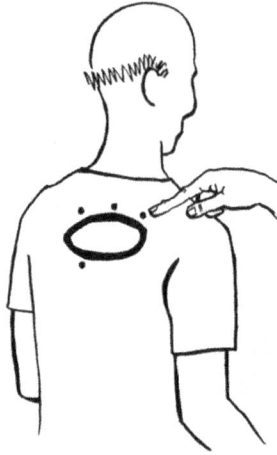

What's for dinner?

People with DSI, especially those who have lost their central vision due to age-related macular degeneration, not only have trouble with faces, they also don't know what is on their plate and where it is. One of the pleasures of dining in and out is visual. We like to know what we are eating and where the things we like (and don't like) are located. By drawing a plate on the back, the communicator can let the diner with DSI know that their chicken is at nine o'clock, the mashed potatoes at six and the peas and beans at twelve. Using a clock face to give locations can also be done on a palm if the back is not accessible or discreet enough.

Emotions

Real-time feedback of the emotional responses of others in the space is socially important. Body language is used to denote emotional context in so many ways: people nodding in agreement or laughing or crying (Lahtinen, Palmer and Lahtinen, 2010). A person with DSI may miss all of this.

If a person with DSI is giving a speech or telling a story, using a repeated up and down movement with the finger communicates: yes, yes, yes, meaning the audience is agreeing with them. If a joke or story makes the audience laugh, by using the hand as though it is clutching a ball moving on and off the upper arm of the person with DSI signifies laughter. This movement should continue as long as the laughter lasts.

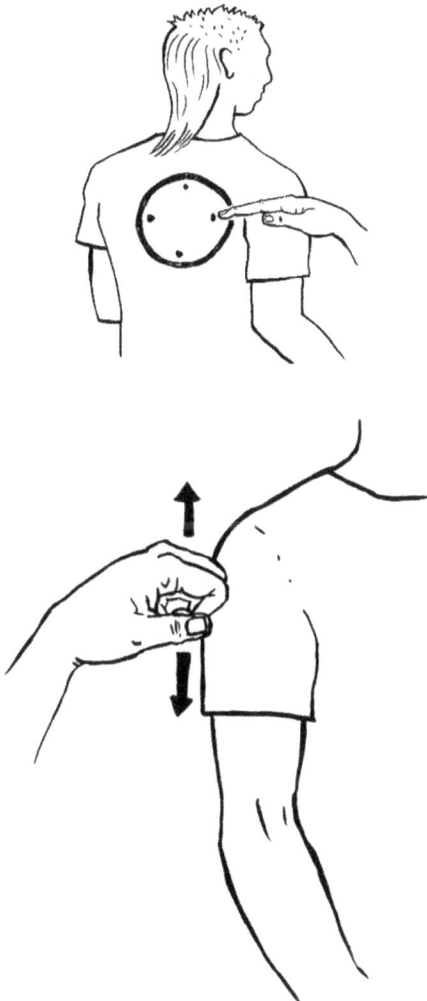

Yes, audience agrees. Audience is laughing.

On the other hand, if the story is amazing or shocking, the communicator starts with all fingertips together on the upper arm then drags them open. This is like an open mouth in shock or awe.

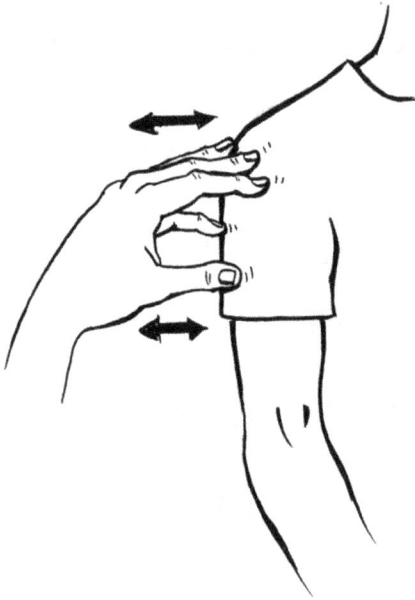

And if the audience is happy or smiling then this is indicated by drawing a smile on the upper arm of the person with DSI. Conversely, if a communicator wishes to convey sadness, then an upside-down smile is drawn. Tears can be demonstrated by using a fingertip to mark out the tracks of tears falling on the upper arm. Note that all these haptices can be applied on the negotiated safe areas of the body, e.g., upper arm, back, or hand.

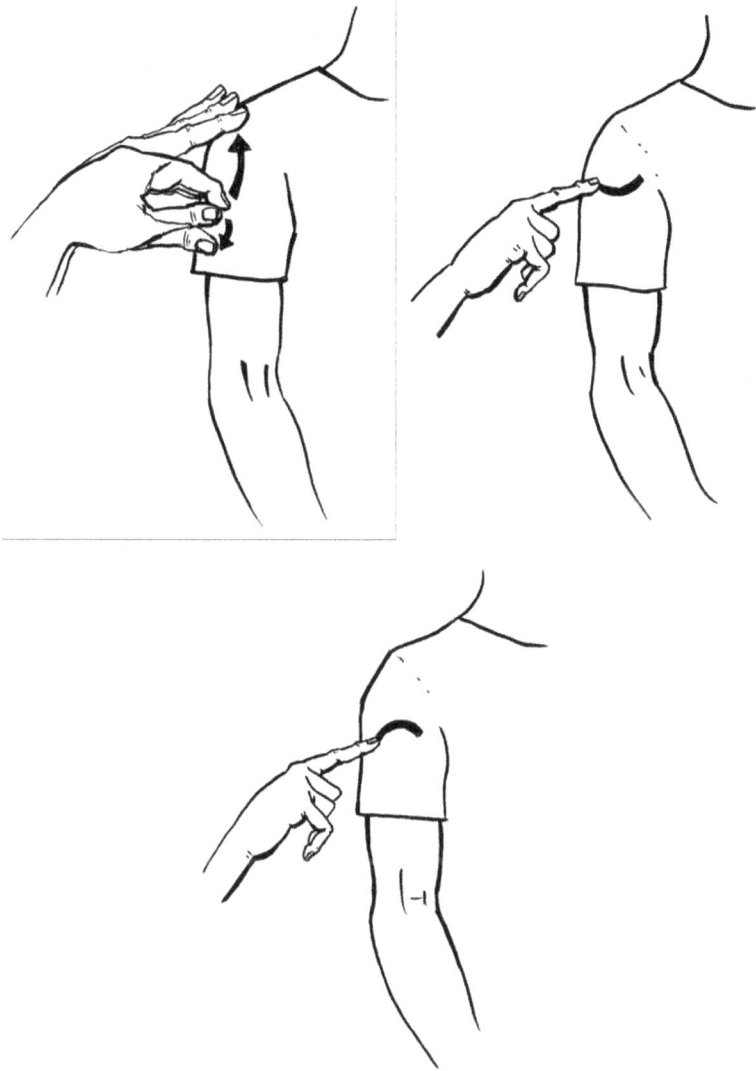

However, if the story, lecture, or speech is boring then this can be signaled by the communicator placing all fingertips together in the center of the upper arm and then opening them outwards like a big yawn.

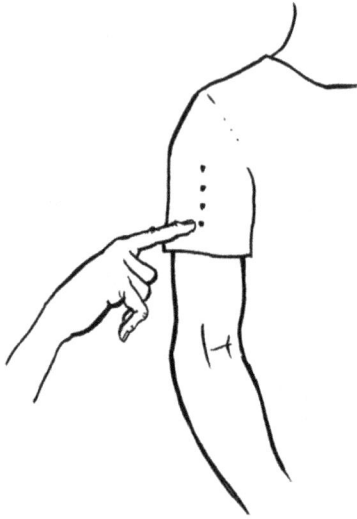

Name sign or "body name"

These were among the earliest developed aspects of social-haptic communication. The use of a "body name" was introduced in the early days to allow a person with DSI "to identify the person coming into their personal space" (Palmer and Lahtinen, 2013, p. 69). Deaf and deafblind communities use name signs that are visual or tactile in nature. This then is a sign that is given to a person that identifies them. A body name sign is likewise given to someone by a person with deafblindness or DSI. A "body name" or tactile name sign needs to be easy to feel and differentiate by the person with DSI. We have used both terms here (name sign or body name) as there may be some who use each term to indicate who people are. There are examples in Chapter 9.

Entering/leaving a space

These haptices were developed early after yes/no, and are really useful to give a person with DSI an idea of who is arriving and who is leaving.

"I am here" is conveyed by the communicator touching the person with DSI on the shoulder. This may be combined with a name sign or body name (if they have one).

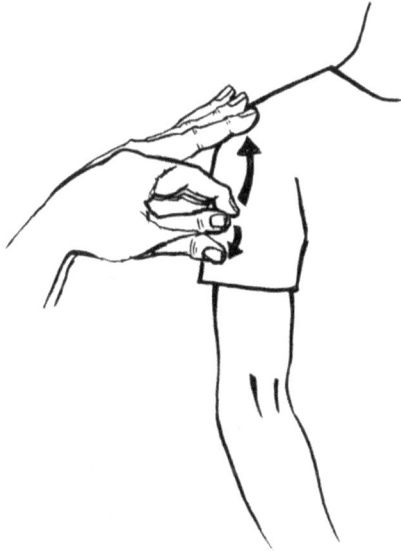

To indicate a person is leaving the space, the communicator can use the flat hand moving (stroking) cross the person's back moving to the direction of leaving.

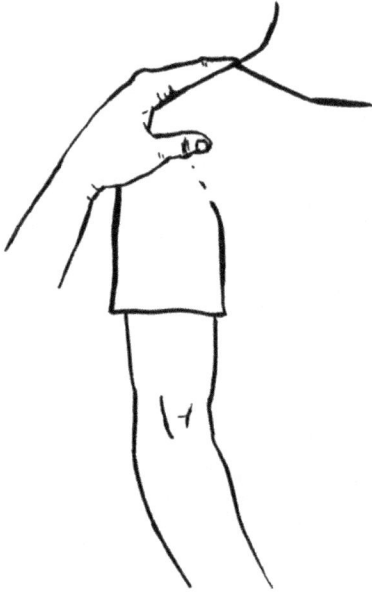

Another way to do this when you can't reach the back, or it is easier to use the arm is for the communicator to make a claw handshape on the upper arm of the person with DSI that moves inwards as in a pinching motion and then away from the body means I am leaving. This is the method used by Author One. This shows how social haptics can be tailored to what an individual needs/wants. The use of the name sign or body name as well as a haptice for I am here or I am going allows the persons with DSI to know who it is that is coming or going.

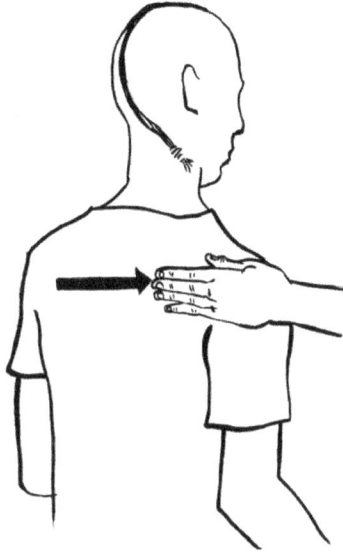

Guiding

UP/DOWN: if person is holding your arm or hand on your shoulder then move your shoulder on that side up (for up) and down (for down) OR

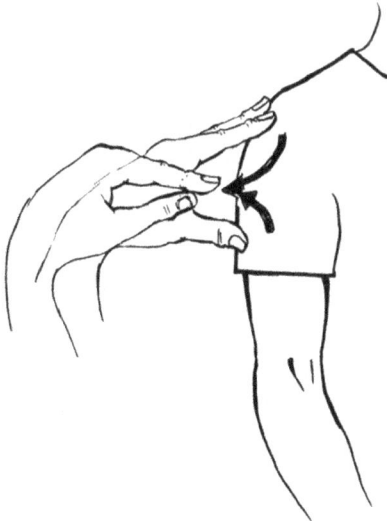

Tap on the hand to indicate a step and move the hand up for a step up and down for step down.

Always STOP before a change in terrain, steps, stairs, curbs, and escalators. This gives the person with DSI time to register the change.

ROUGH GROUND/CHANGE OF WALKING SURFACE

Fingertips on upper hand moving up and down randomly to indicate uneven surface.

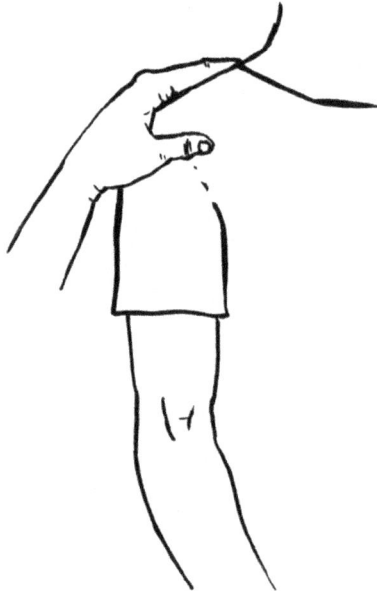

ESCALATOR

Make a chopping motion on the arm or hand followed by moving the hand/arm downwards or upwards to the indicated direction of travel.

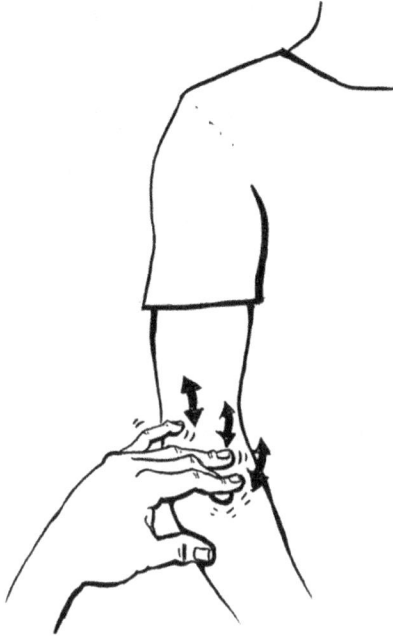

Health

Nowhere is social haptics more useful as a quick messaging system than in healthcare. It does not reduce or eliminate the need for structured and individual communication support for important communication that facilitates shared decision making for patients with disability. Where touch messaging works best is as shortcut haptices for what is about to happen, particularly in hospitals.

Author One has found that the distress and anxiety provoked by unexpected events such as injections is reduced or eliminated entirely by the use of a touch message. Note that social haptics in this setting depend on having the haptices not only learned by the patient but documented in ways that can be shared with health staff at the times needed. This is where health and social care professionals and students can help people with DSI manage some of the difficulties of an admission.

Routine observations are a predictable part of any hospital stay but can cause confusion, distress, and even combativeness when a patient doesn't know what is happening. One of Author One's research participants says, "I just push them away". This is not helpful as staff may misconstrue or interpret this as aggression.

So, this is where touch messaging can be helpful: saving time, reducing distress, and simply letting patients with a communication disability know what is going to happen. In emergencies, even just using Yes and No allows patients to ask questions, "do I need an operation" and staff can say "Yes" by touch message while awaiting more formal communication support. Again, we use the work of Lahtinen and Palmer adapted for the Australian context.

Please note that social-haptic communication is not a language and would not be an effective or equitable method to gain informed consent. You will need to pivot to a language-based method which may or may not include some haptices as needed.

Haptices for health

*   Yes/No

    Yes: Closed fist moving in a nodding motion up and down

    OR

    Finger moving up and down the arm, or up and down on the palm of the hand.

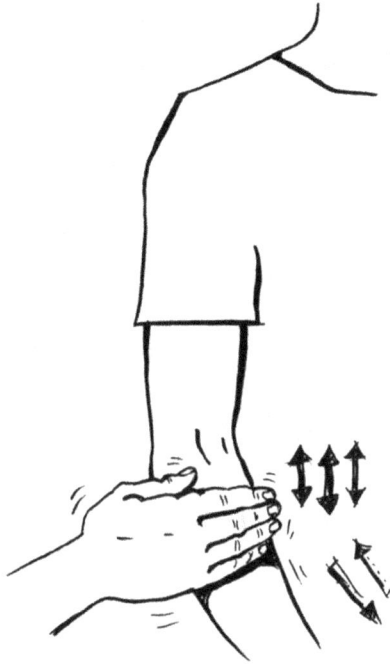

No: Closed fist moving in a shaking motion left-right-left-right OR

Fingers doing a rubbing out motion on the upper arm or the palm of the hand.

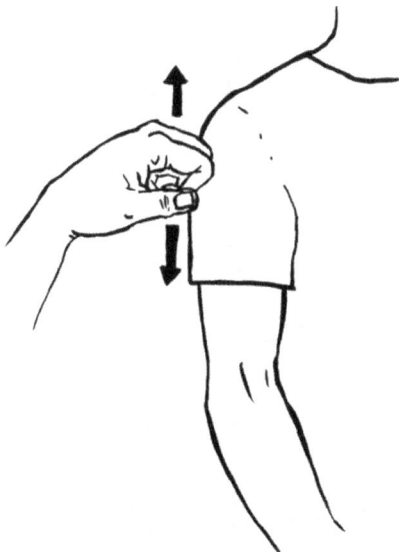

- Emergency. Draw a large 'X' on the back with blade of the hand or finger (press firmly). This means come with me now and I will explain later.

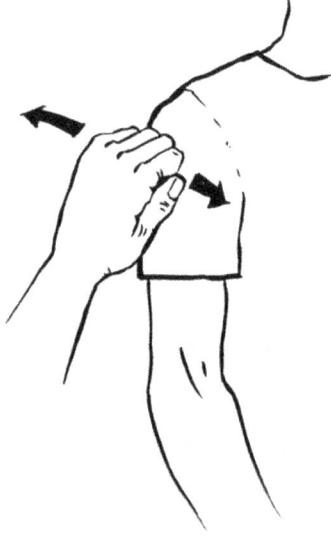

- Doctor/nurse: Use the fingertip of the index finger and draw a medical cross on the upper arm or hand.

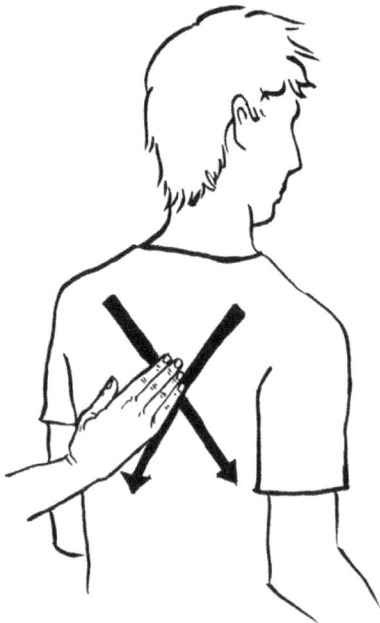

- I'm here: Hand on shoulder light to moderate pressure.

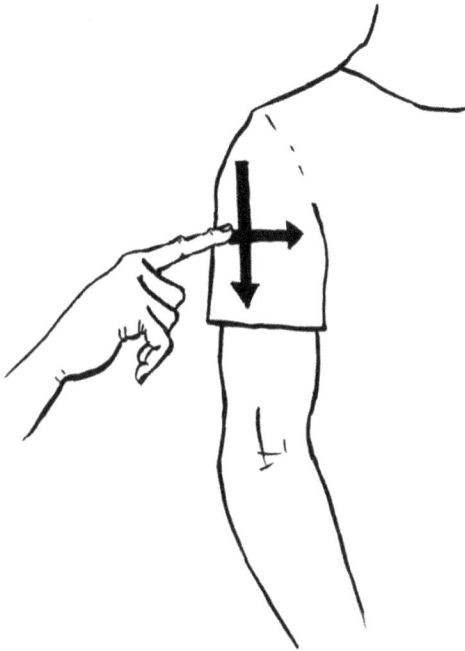

- Blood pressure check (and also observations): Use hand to form a "cuff" around the upper arm (in the manner of a blood pressure cuff) and squeeze gently.

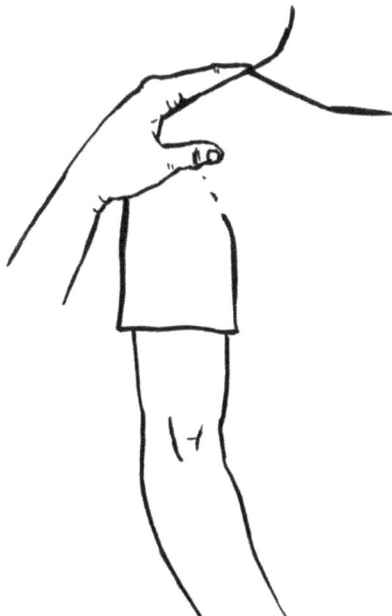

- Pain and where on the body: Claw handshape on the part of the body. A doctor might press a clawed hand on the abdomen and then draw a question mark on the upper arm. This would signify asking: Do you have pain here?

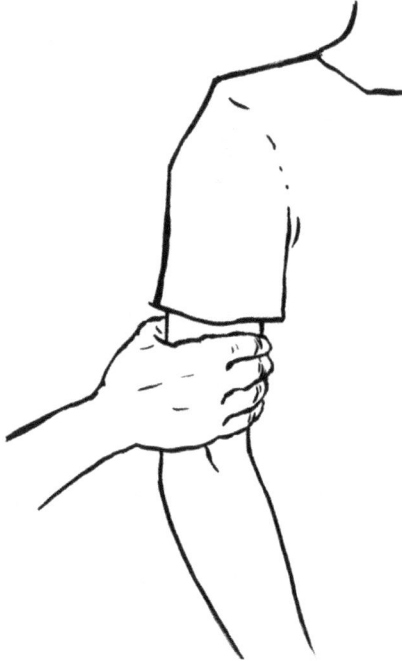

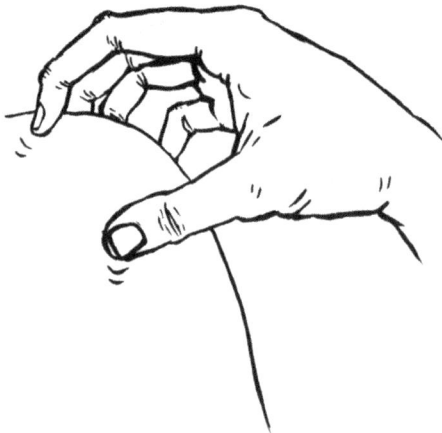

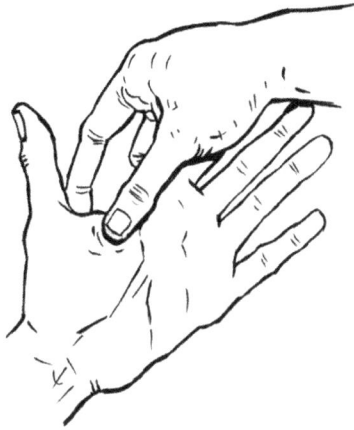

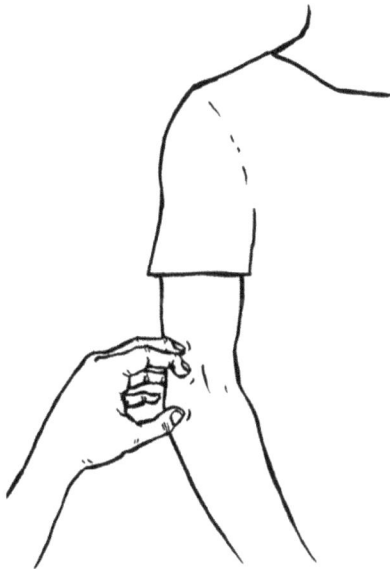

- Injection: Lightly grasp/pinch with thumb and index finger the webbing between the person's thumb and forefinger. Then move finger to the part of the body where the needle will go, e.g., fingertip for finger prick; back of the hand for an intravenous drip; crook of the elbow for a blood test or drip; or the muscle of the upper arm for a vaccination for example.

- Tablets to take: The communicator uses thumb and forefinger to make a pecking motion on the palm of the person with DSI's hand. This simulates the picking up of pills or tablets and swallowing them.

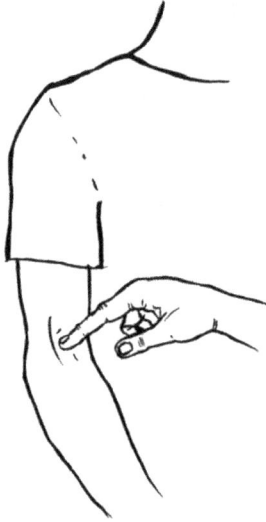

- Are you ok?: Three ways of doing this.

  1. Thumbs up and grab the thumb or 2. Smiling emotion haptice on the upper arm with a question mark drawn on the upper arm. You can also just draw a question mark on the upper arm.

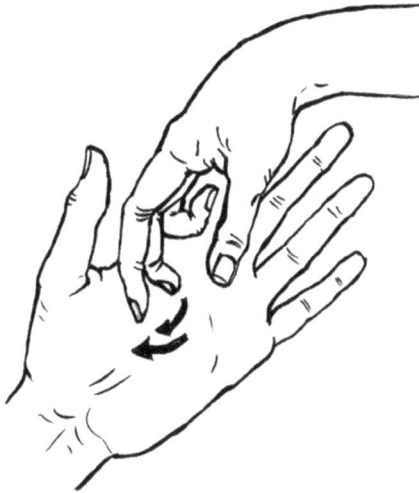

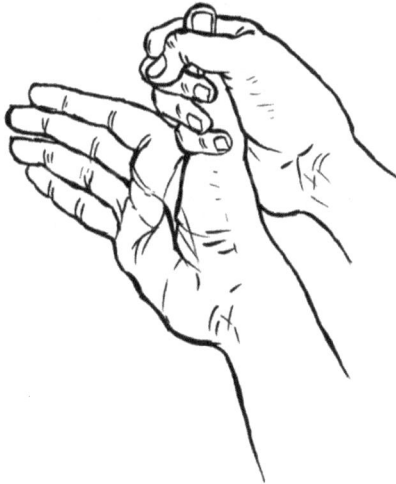

- Stay calm, stay still. Hand on the shoulder with some firm but gentle pressure.

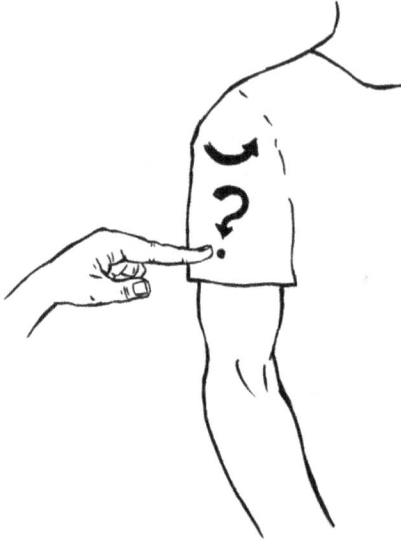

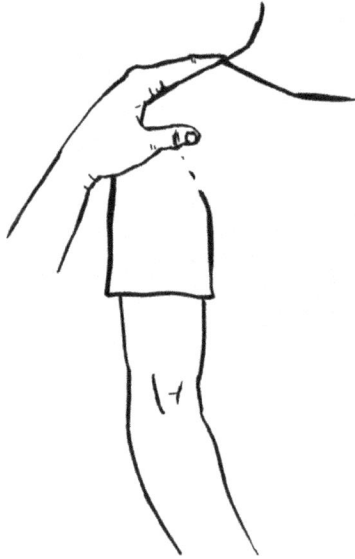

Documenting systems, signals, messages, and haptices

This is of critical importance. Once you have a social communication framework, people with DSI have the ability to generate new tactile haptices for new needs.

An example from Author One's experience is that at university meetings, conferences, and seminars etc. there are often technical glitches getting Zoom going, PowerPoints up, and microphones to work. It was realized that a tactile message was needed to say there is a delay while organizers or lecturers sort out a technical "glitch". So, a haptice was made to signal this: The communicator moves the fingers randomly around the palm or upper arm. So, it becomes important that these are included in one's arsenal and communicated to others in the support team.

Whatever signs, messages, signals, haptices, and alphabets that an individual with DSI (or any other communication disability) needs, uses, and invents, need to be documented as there is no general social or health worker awareness of these methods. We suggest using:

> Communication book where descriptions of all signs etc. in use can be recorded. This will end up acting like a small dictionary with the vocabulary and shortcut messages;
> Hard copy sheets of these signs, signals, haptices, and alphabets, laminated, if possible, to make them more durable. These should go with the person to each healthcare visit or hospital stay. The healthcare haptices fit on a single page (back and front);

Where possible, record the touch messages used, e.g., as photos in a folder in your smartphone;

Ensure that family friends, GP, and allied health workers are all informed and get a chance to practice the messages with the person with DSI; and

Don't forget new support workers need to learn tactile messaging systems used by the client. Make time for current and new supports to learn and take-home information sheets.

Conclusion

What we need now is more dissemination of social-haptic communication. We need more research on how best to integrate teaching and learning with older people with DSI. We know older people learn differently. We know older people with DSI may not be able to listen and look at the same time. We know older people have different residuals, so learning is very individual. These are factors to consider when deciding which methods and systems to learn.

There are also many other population groups who can benefit from tactile messaging systems like social-haptic communication such as those with: single sensory impairments; younger people and children with single and dual sensory impairment; anyone with an intellectual disability or traumatic brain injury (sensory loss is a common, often undiagnosed feature of both these); or anyone with a communication disability, temporary or permanent.

So, we need to arm ourselves and those who need touch messaging to understand what is about to happen. Health haptics from social-haptic communication are beneficial for: staff and wider society as improved patient experiences are strongly associated with better health and well-being outcomes (Sutherland et al., 2017); patients who understand what is happening are more likely to be compliant so procedures, tests, and observations are less time costly; patient compliance and safety is improved (Slade et al., 2015) and money is saved by the fewer readmissions and representations in health services (Slade et al., 2015). In short, better communication leads to better experiences (Lang, 2012) and better social participation (Palmer and Lahtinen, 2013). Social-haptic communication can be a part of a wholistic support for those living with DSI. Chapter 9 will look at other components of communication support that work well with or without social-haptic communication to provide context, meaning, and inclusion for those older people with DSI. Following that we look at preparing people with DSI for hospital admissions, emergencies, and disasters. In Chapter 11, we will show you a case story in which it can be seen how social-haptic communication can fit in with sign shortcuts, names, signs, and "body name" and manual alphabets to create a collection of potential communication supports for older people living with DSI and their families.

9
Living better

Communication 3: Name signs, print on palm, fingerspelling, and personalized systems

Introduction

Social haptics is not the only touch messaging system people with dual sensory impairment (DSI)—together with their families and carers—can use to supplement communication. We now look at some easy to learn and remember ways of communicating words and messages: name signs, print on palm, manual alphabets, and personalized messaging systems.

Name signs

This is what we think of as the fun part of tactile messaging. It is so helpful to have signals that identify our important people, so they can let us know who is there. These can be derived from tactile signs, manual alphabet, or tactile representations of special characteristics of individuals. Individuals should be aware that the name sign devised for them has to work from the person with DSI's perspective. So, it's not something others without DSI get to choose and enforce. There has to be significance and easy recognition by the person with DSI. Name signs are different for each individual so if there are two Marys or Johns then a different name sign is given to each.

Author One will present the example from their family, friendship, work, and support groups:

Author One: A flick by the right index and thumb on the left thumb (like the sign for champagne in Auslan). Obviously, Author One likes champagne;

Author Two: Fingers "marching" on the upper arm to signify Scottish dancing. Author Two is from Scotland;

Partner: Touching the wedding band on the left hand;

Child 1: Writing their initials on the upper arm (they also write for a living);

Child 2: Their first initial on the upper arm;

Child 3: The manual alphabet of their first initial on the left hand;

Daughter-in-law: Manual alphabet first initial on the upper arm (works in combination with Child 2 to indicate the two of them);

Friend: An Eiffel tower shape up the arm;

Friend: The Auslan sign for airplane up the arm (this person is a great traveler);

Friend: Uses "marching" fingers on the shoulder (so different location to previous marching fingers);

Friend: A manual alphabet T followed by one finger on the palm to signify Twin One;

Friend: Touching left index fingertip (manual alphabet for E) and going down into a finger on the palm for L in the manual alphabet;

Friend: A hooked finger around the little finger on the left hand (sign of S in the manual alphabet);

Friend: Right hand of the friend clasps the left wrist in the manner of a bangle (which is a favorite accessory of the friend);

Friend: Draw a smile on the upper arm followed by two three fingered taps (as in the letter M in the manual alphabet). This derives from this person being a happy mother of several children; and

Friend: Random strokes on the upper arm with a finer touch (simulating paint brush strokes, as this friend is an artist).

Name signs are very personal and often tell a story of their own. They are also useful for knowing who is talking to you, especially for those who have lost the ability to see faces as in age related macular degeneration (the commonest cause of low vision in older age). Name signs can be combined with social haptics as described in Chapter 7: Living better: Communication 1. For example, going around a bridge table, a family meal table, or in a restaurant. A communication partner can draw the table on the back and indicate where the person with DSI is sitting, then go around using name signs to indicate where known friends, family, colleagues, and peers are sitting. Manual alphabets can be used to introduce and locate those who don't have a name sign assigned to them.

Print on palm

This can be an easy way to convey short or urgent messages by printing capital letters onto the palm (or arm, leg, or face even). One contributor to Stoffel's *Deafblind Reality* (2011) describes how during a neurological illness only her cheeks remained as a communication conduit. The family and hospital staff could print short messages using their finger onto the patient's cheek. For a participant in our research, Barbara in her residential aged-care facility (where none of the staff have bothered to learn a manual alphabet), staff printing on her hand or forearm is the only communication she gets. But, as with manual alphabets, good spelling is essential for meaning making as Barbara notes that poor spelling is common among the staff where she is and "bad spelling is the same as no communication". But print on palm is a good strategy that staff in aged care, healthcare, and hospitals can try in an emergency.

Fingerspelling

Social-haptic communication isn't a language and while for beginners it can be very slow, manual alphabets allow you to compose whole sentences with fingerspelling. Author One's family and assistants fingerspell using Australian sign language's deafblind manual alphabet. Fingerspelling is frequently used to contextualize conversations and correct misunderstandings. As an example, a single word spelled out, e.g., "holidays" can give context to a conversation going on around them when snippets are being heard but the subject remains elusive.

In Australia, many older people aging with DSI have learned this communication method as the prime language. Auslan (Australian sign language) was not formally recognized by the Australian government until 1987. Teaching d/Deafblind children in the early decades of the twentieth century relied on the tactile manual alphabet where one person spells letters of the alphabet on to the other's palm and fingers. In good news for older Australians with DSI, many schools from 2023 will begin learning Auslan and this includes the manual alphabet.

We could learn a tactile sign language such as hand-over-hand Australian sign language and a few of us do. But, as with any language, it takes a few years to get vocabulary and fluency. In the meantime, fingerspelling by our communication partners can decrease tension, correct misassumptions, and convey information.

Thus, fingerspelling is an easy to learn system of denoting the letters of the alphabet on the palm and hand. Sometimes, we haven't got the subject or detail wrong, instead we have no idea of the topic under discussion. Knowing the subject allows us to contextualize and contribute meaningfully and be included. Author One will draw a question mark on the communication partner's hand if they are clueless as to the content of conversations. The partner then fingerspells the information. They find this a more peaceful process than asking, "What are we talking about?" all the time.

People with DSI (or hearing loss alone) can enjoy a discreet spelling on the hand instead of repeated shouting of words, phrases, or instructions. Fingerspelling comes in handy for example at movies or theaters. For example, having "s-t-a-r-t" when a movie, play, or musical event is beginning so that we stop talking and take our seats. Or, the alphabet can be used to signal who is talking to you if there is no name sign for that person, e.g., R-O-Y. Using the deafblind alphabet also enables contextual words to be given, e.g., the subject of a discussion or if a concept or word has been misunderstood, e.g., "I am going to get a coffee" was misunderstood by Author One as "I am going to get a puppy". By fingerspelling c-o-f-f-e-e, the confusion is cleared up straightaway.

But fingerspelling effectiveness relies on correct spelling by the communication partner. If a word is misspelled it is the same as no communication. If spelling is an issue, pivot to a different method. Communication partners often worry they are not fast enough with the manual alphabet but usually we recipients are very slow. This is new to us too, and we have to concentrate very hard on what's being spelled. It is important to use firm pressure as it is very common for all older people to have less sensation in the fingers, and some may have conditions that result in peripheral neuropathies. Find the right pressure level for your person with DSI. Partners need to leave a discernible gap between spelling each word otherwise they all run into each other and make no sense.

Deafblind manual alphabet (Australian)
A

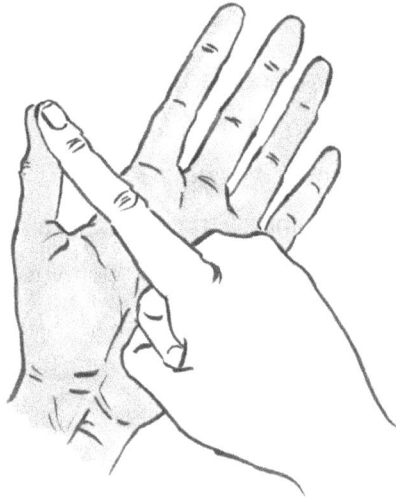

B

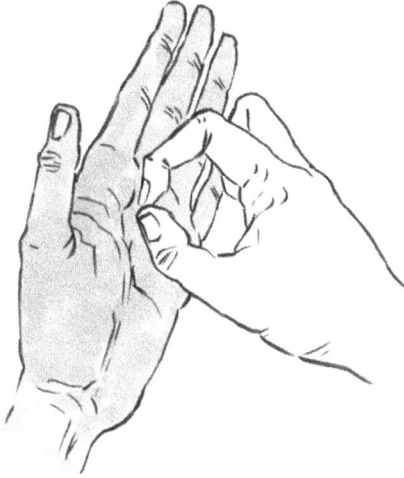

C

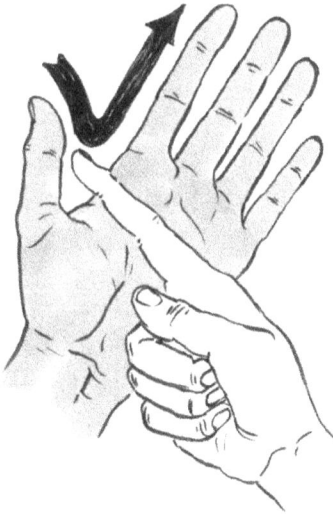

D

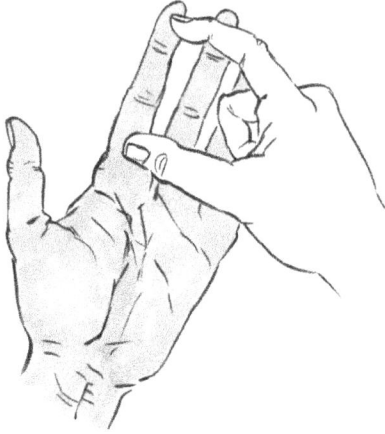

E

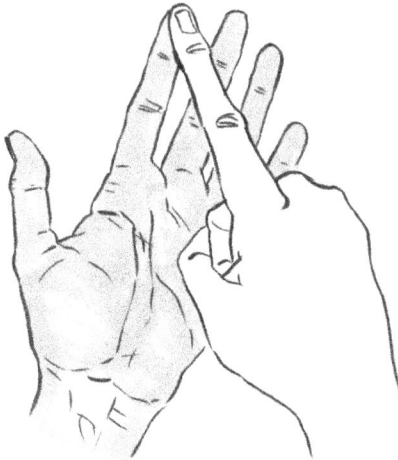

F

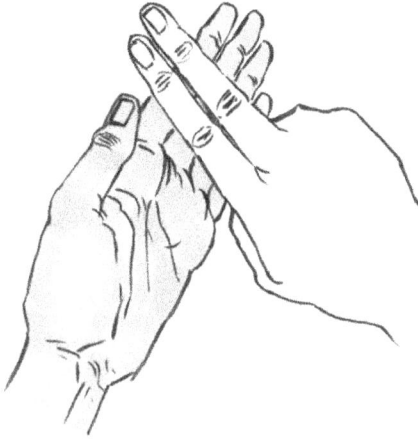

G

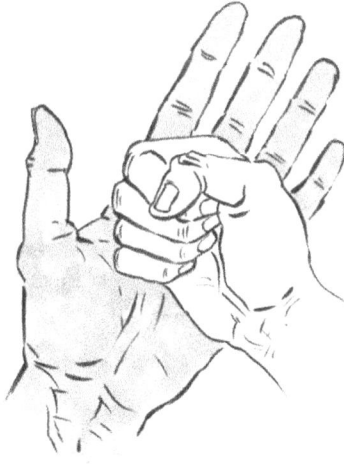

H

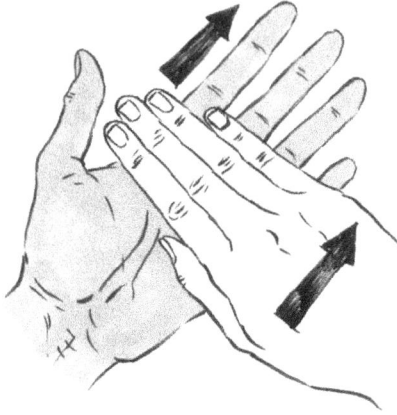

I

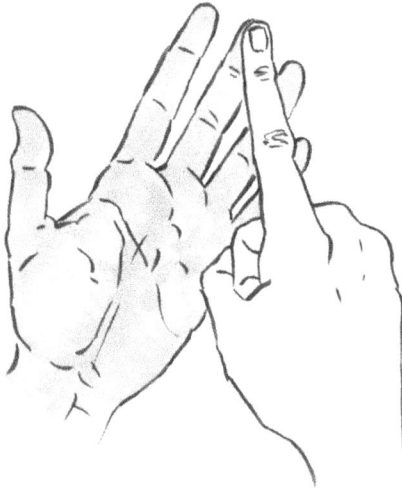

J

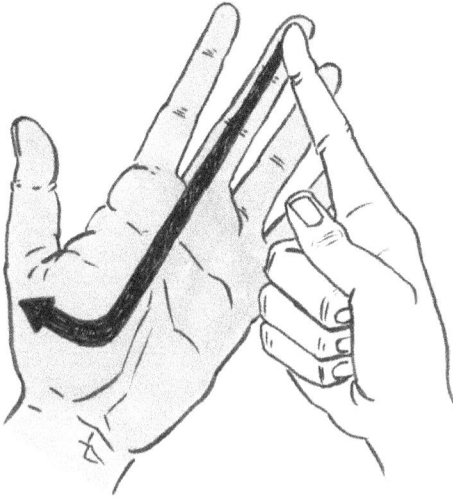

K

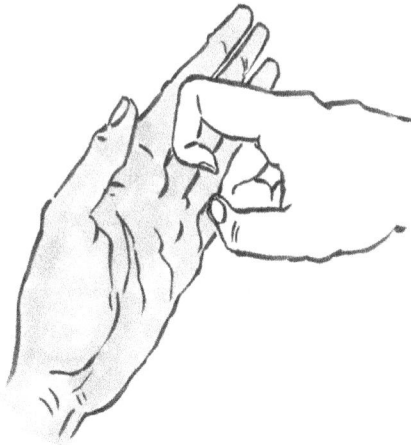

L

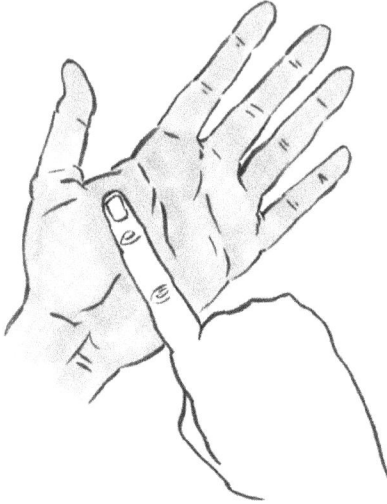

M

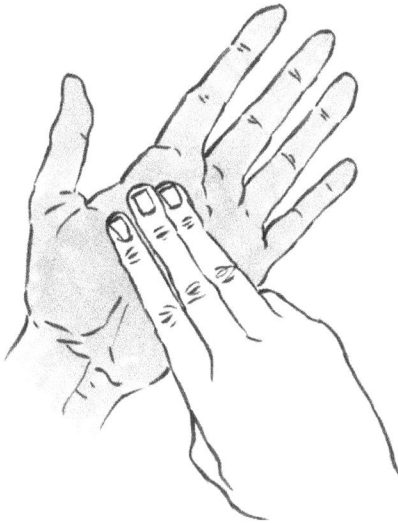

N

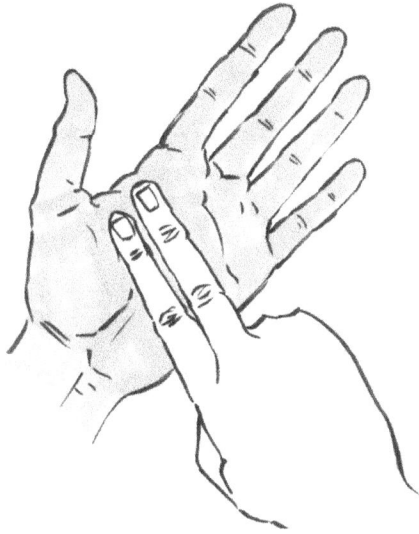

O

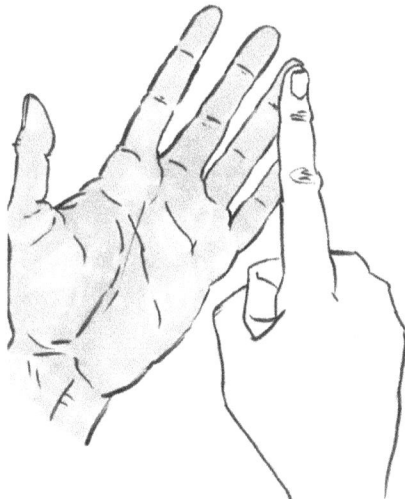

P

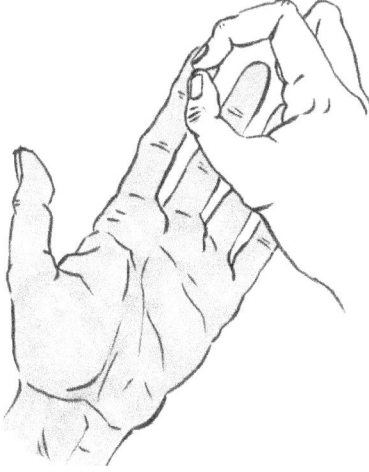

Q

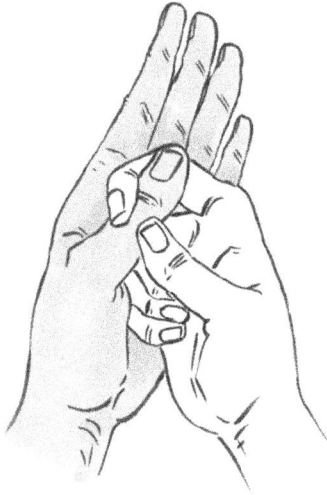

R

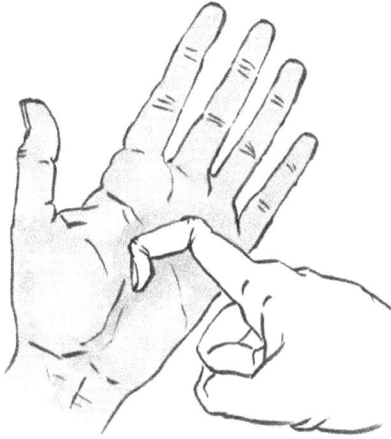

S

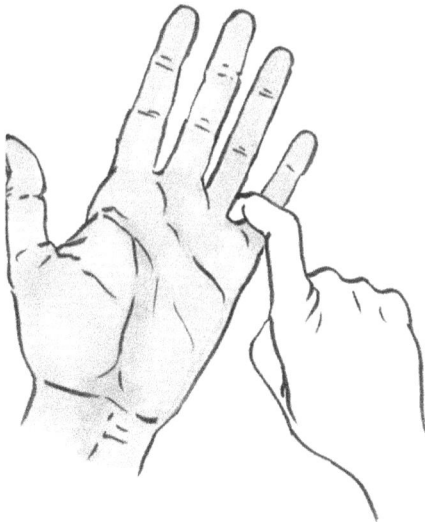

T

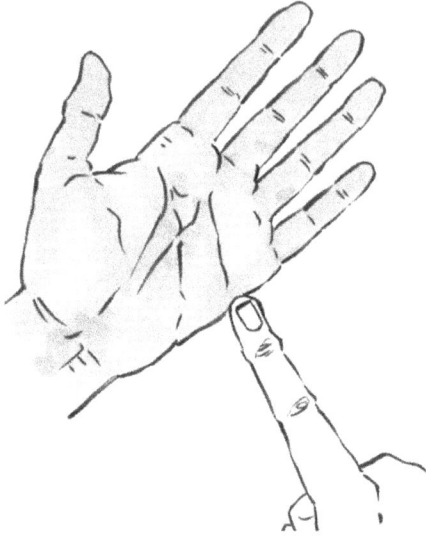

U

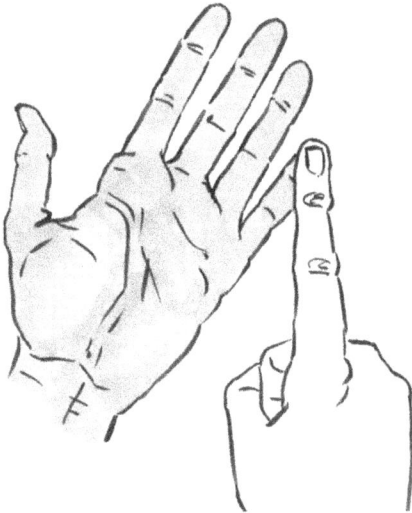

V

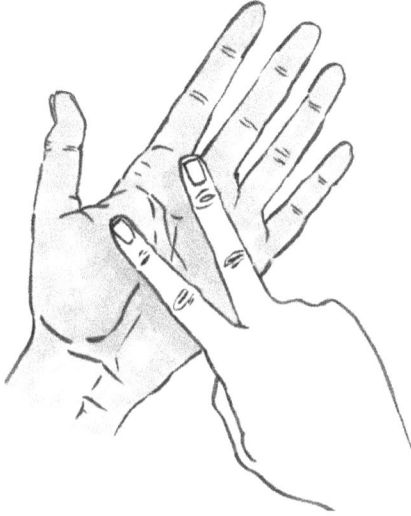

W

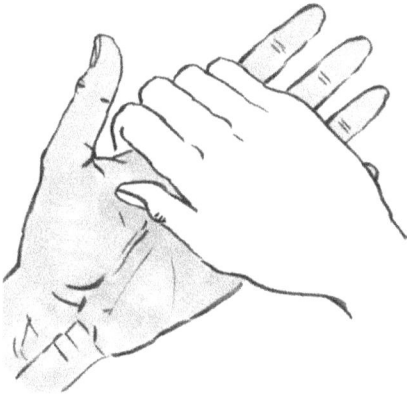

X

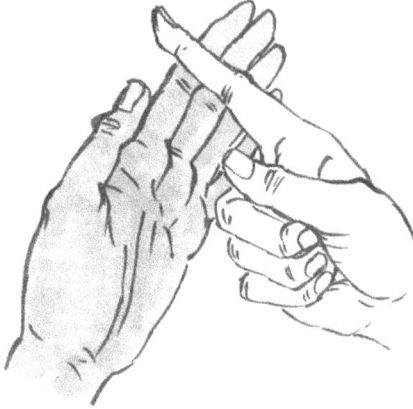

Y

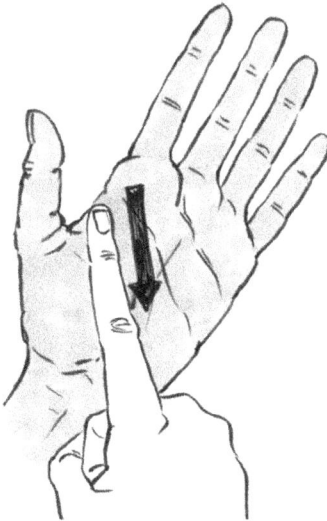

z

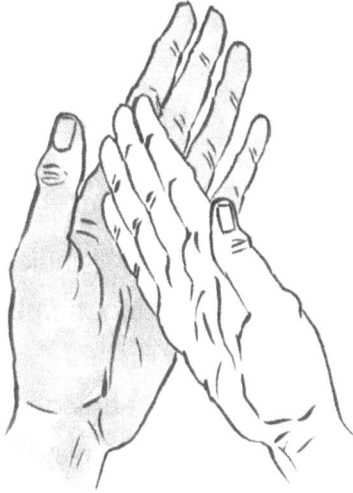

Links to other countries' deafblind manual alphabets

Australian: www.deafblindinformation.org.au/living-with-deafbl
indness/deafblind-communication/deafblind-manual-
alphabet/

British: https://actiondeafness.org.uk/learning-the-deafblind-man
ual-alphabet/

American:www.afb.org/about-afb/history/online-museums/anne-
sullivan-miracle-worker/formative-years/manual-alphabet

Swedish: www.deafblind.com/swedisma.html

Norwegian: www.deafblind.com/norwayma.html

Greek: www.deafblind.com/greecema.html

German: www.deafblind.com/germama.html

Russian: www.deafblind.com/russima.html

Spanish: www.deafblind.com/spain.html

Personalized, idiosyncratic, and other messaging methods

Developing touch messages for an individual's interests and needs may be needed where existing touch messaging systems fail or lack the vocabulary. An example is touch messages for playing bridge, e.g., for one older person with DSI, their support person came up with a tactile system to indicate the bids: with different signals for each suit (touching thumb for hearts, index finger for clubs etc.) and print on palm for the number of tricks bid. No trumps were signified by a rubbing out motion on the palm. All players used extra-large print playing cards (available from the Vision Australia shop) so that accessibility belonged to everyone and the participant felt included.

Another participant had their own idiosyncratic series of touch messages for short cut communications but this was only used (and known) by the immediate family. New support workers were taught the system. Problems arose, however, when they went to hospital or family were suddenly unavailable with unfamiliar support people struggling to communicate. This is why documenting the signs, taking photos, making drawings, and then writing them out in a communication book that can go to hospital, on healthcare visits, and travel with the persons with DSI is important.

Document all the communication methods used

It is really important for people using idiosyncratic touch and/or other messaging to document these both electronically and in hard copy. It is also crucial that ALL methods are documented and described. We strongly advise making a few laminated sheets so that you are "ready" if you ever have to go to a health center or hospital for example. Taking photos of signals and tactile on-body messaging and keeping them in a folder on a smart phone is a sensible strategy as these can be shown to healthcare professionals or new support workers. They should also be printed out and laminated, if possible, so that there is a hard copy that can be immediately used.

We also suggest a TOP FIVE (Top 5) communication methods approach listing for important conversations, e.g., health and hospital. List your preferred modes of communication so that those communicating with you can PIVOT to another method if one isn't working. As an example, Author One's top five are: Use hearing aids for face-to-face oral communication; use speech to text app (Otter AI on smart phone or tablet); manual alphabet (sheet in the going to hospital bag for attaching to bedside); and finally, if all else fails, contacting Author One's partner on their mobile phone.

If you use social-haptic communication, health haptic communication, idiosyncratic messaging, or manual alphabet, include copies of these so that wherever you go, whenever needed, people can communicate short messages and words to help you work out what is going on. Personal messaging sheets should also include:

- Touch messages our family and carers use;
- Touch and other signals our health professionals can use with us;

- Alternative communication modes, e.g., pen and paper, thick Texta, whiteboard, speech to text, text to speech, and so on;
- Settling techniques family and carers use with us when we are anxious;
- Information on devices we use to assist communication and plain language instructions on how to use these, as not everyone is up to date or familiar with every device. Instructions should also advise how to recharge and how to change batteries; and
- Top five communication methods listed so that a pivot can be made when one method no longer works.

Conclusion

We have canvassed a few of the tactile messaging systems in use in Australia with links to the manual alphabet from other countries as well. We also advise that family/carer dyads and groups will likely develop their own systems that are personal and specific. Both authors strongly advise documenting these, to have this crucial communication information to hand when going to healthcare visits and hospital. In Chapter 10, we will look at strategies to manage healthcare and hospitalizations so that older people living with DSI have a better chance of knowing what is going on and participating in their own care decisions. Chapter 10 will show how we can pull all these strategies together to make life happier, healthier, and safer for an older person with DSI.

10
Being prepared

Hospital admission and emergency planning

Introduction

There are many ways that health professionals, practitioners, and families can help people with dual sensory impairment (DSI). We have looked at communication and ways to promote better living with DSI. We can also help patients and clients learn new ways and new technologies, we can pivot to another method, we can certify conditions, and provide access to social care supports. We can all collaborate and support older people with DSI to live better and plan better for emergencies. A large gap exists around hospital and emergency preparedness. Here, we present information (with a real case example) firstly, to prepare for hospitalizations, and secondly, for emergencies and disasters.

Preparing people with DSI for health and hospital encounters

Preparation is important for health and hospital encounters. People living with DSI can help themselves be better prepared.

But we/they need their families, health and social care professionals, and practitioners to help curate and collect what is needed. Having our important information at hand, both electronically and in a hard copy, saves time and reduces communication stress with our health providers. If the admitting doctor is spending time trying to work out what those little white tablets we take are called, they aren't focusing on telling us what we need to know about what will happen next. Staff won't have time to answer our questions if we don't have a clear method of communication/s that can be used.

This means encouraging patients/clients to have their up-to-date information in two separate spaces, as an online version and hard copy. This information should be collected, placed in a bag or folder, and kept somewhere easy to find during an emergency. Health and social care workers can be proactive in ensuring changes in conditions and treatments, and new conditions are entered into health information folders. This is additional to the electronic health record as it is patient controlled. This can include information about health, communication needs, care plans, and plain language information for managing communication devices. Patients can use the Top 5 or My Health Matters Folder to help create this resource.

Here is an example of a real going-to-hospital kit for an older person with DSI with some commentaries about how its different components are experienced in the real hospital world. My own going-to-hospital kit comes in two forms: information on my smartphone and within a turquoise-blue cloth bag hanging on the back of my bedroom door. This has large sequins on it, so I am able to tell it apart from other cloth bags. I am late to the hospital kit party; while I knew academically that these are such sensible preparations, I was not motivated to actually do the information gathering it required until the pandemic struck Australia's shores in March 2020. Covid-19 made me realize that, if and when I went to hospital, I could not have the reassuring presence of a communication partner to bring things in because I needed them to advocate for me (except by phone). My experience has been that younger staff go for speech-to-text and older ones use the whiteboard or pen and paper. Basically, keep a list of your most important apps because staff are there for the essentials and basics. If you have hearing (lucky, lucky you) and listen to music, include earbuds and playlist information because staff may be able to set you up with the sounds you love if you are too unwell to do so yourself. Preload audio books if this is something you can enjoy.

Duly motivated, I began assembling:

- Information on my smartphone, with a hard copy for the cloth bag kit. This includes emergency information, health information, card numbers, photos of my prescriptions (the doctor in me prefers this to photos of labels on tablet packets), vaccine certificates, and so on. One day, I hope that the Department of Health will have a care passport app (with hard-copy contents for the cloth bag) so there is a systematized way to gather this information that is sanctioned, consistent, and encouraged by health authorities, and which staff are familiar with. Many disabled people's organizations have advocated for system wide healthcare passports, e.g., Julian's Key but the departments of health have yet to engage (Queensland Government, 2022). Some health professionals have clinical document architecture files that can be shared to patient smartphones, but I am not that organized at present. I have my allergies, health, and disability information in the emergency access part of my phone;

- A cloth bag, hardware, hard copies of information, and laminated deafblind manual alphabet plus printed sheets to spare. It is sad but true that hospitals are places where things are lost, especially patient belongings and printed information, so I have several copies. In an ideal world, I would have a pad with tear-off sheets, but that day is not here (yet);

- Social-haptic communication. As observed earlier, I have found this to be both reassuring and informative in practice. There are enough words to tell me who is there (doctor/ nurse) and what they want to do (give me medicine to take or an injection in my arm), but I have a sheet with the touch messages I use and a description of how they are performed. If I am lucky, my interpreter, a family member, or my support worker may visit and demonstrate them in person, in situ. If I am not too unwell, I can show staff too. The ones that are the most useful for me are a touch on the shoulder (I am here) followed by a cross drawn on shoulder or hand (I am a doctor or nurse), and a cuff of thumb and index finger on the upper arm to indicate blood pressure (so reassuring in the early hours of the morning when I am woken for observations). I use this cuff signal for the whole group of temperature, pulse, blood pressure, respiration rate, oxygen level, wound inspection, drain inspection, and so on. For me, it sends the message that predictable things are going to happen. I also like the injection touch signal of a light pinch on the injection site (such as the fingers, or crook of the elbow, or abdomen). The surgeon can also grasp my thumb to tell me it all went well. These touch messages are combined with finger spelling for more complicated messaging such as going for an X-ray. This is not a language but a touch messaging system, so it is easy for staff to learn and I ask for both charts to be taped near my bed. We will look at touch messaging systems in the next chapter in more detail. But whatever system/s we use, they should be documented so that staff can learn and use them;

- A thick pen and notebook may also work as a communication tool (I have a little residual vision). I use a Pentel Sign Pen because it does not bleed and I am able to see it, whereas I cannot see biros or thinner felt-tip markers. I need more than one communication method; for example, if I were to have cataract surgery, or I am unwell or not wearing glasses, pen and paper will fail me. One communication method cannot be relied upon in all settings. The staff need to print in big letters, too. This is written on the front of the front of the notebook;

- A small whiteboard and suitable markers. My support worker found these in a two-dollar shop, and they have been brilliant for those wishing to communicate in hospital with me. Sometimes, I just need a word or phrase to understand and contextualize what is going on, such as "Doctor Smith", "Nurse Jones", "physio", or "new drip" (meaning a cannula is going to be inserted or re-sited);

- An orange silicone wristband saying "I AM DEAFBLIND". In fact, I have about three in my bag just in case I am forced to take it off, such as when going to theater. The last time I went to hospital, the nurse gave up trying to remove it before theater and simply covered it with tape, similar to how wedding rings are taped. Then she laboriously wrote in pen "I am Deafblind" on the tape. I did not object because something is better than nothing, even if the process made little sense. These have been the best supports because, wherever I go, they identify me to staff as a patient needing communication support, and they remind the staff at every encounter, every shift, every day and night. They are portable, cheap, and effective;

- Chargers for my iPad and smartphone. These are spare chargers that live in my going-to-hospital bag. Seriously, devices do not work when out of power or battery, and waiting a night or day for a cord to power up a communication device is not good for my anxiety levels;

- A sheet with the common apps I use (I am not a techno whiz so there are a great many that younger or more tech-savvy people know of and use). I have instructions on what each app holds and how to access it:
  - The health app has the most important health details such as allergies, main conditions, and medications;
  - The Kindle app holds my books and is set to my preferred (very large) font style;
  - The Notes app can be used for speech-to-text—it is on dark mode and set to large font, so it is ready to go for my particular needs; and
  - The on-screen keyboard can also be used as an aid.

- A list in big letters saying "BRING IPAD, BRING IPHONE, BRING HEARING AIDS". It is not sensible, for the planet or the pocket, to have duplicate devices; and

- Hearing aid batteries in a clear Ziplock bag. Two packets. Last, but emphatically not the least important, I have a sheet (plus copies) with information on my sensory losses. It is longer than most staff have time for, but I want to make the most of every opportunity to educate and inform with less "wear and tear" on myself.

Emergency and disaster preparedness

It's really important we all have conversations around emergencies and disasters. Large areas of Australia have been and presently are, impacted by climate disasters and we all lived through Covid-19 lockdowns. In some communities more than 20 percent of the residents are older. Since sensory impairment rates are high in older people (see chapter 2), they all need to talk with their partners, families, and support networks about how they will manage in an emergency.

The largest gap in emergency planning and disaster preparedness is around individuals in the community. Everyone and everybody benefits from better emergency preparedness: Older people generally and older people with DSI, people with disabilities, carers, families, children, young people, First Nations peoples, homeless, people from cultural and linguistically diverse communities, people living in public housing, people living in group homes, people living on their own, people with chronic conditions and/or serious health issues, people who need individualized supports to manage daily life, and people living in rural and remote areas. So, pretty much nearly everyone and everybody can be at risk in an emergency and therefore, we should all be having conversations about our preparedness and making solid plans.

A good disaster plan helps keep people independent, maintains health and well-being and reduces the need for emergency help. A good disaster plan allows us to shelter-in-place safely and/or to evacuate early as needed. A good disaster plan helps carers and families as well as emergency service workers know what supports are needed and how to communicate better. Good disaster preparedness can reduce the burden on emergency services (leaving them free to save other lives), and helps local supports and councils plan their community responses better.

Health and social care professionals can also assist older people with DSI (and indeed all their patients and clients) by having an emergency planning conversation and collaborating with a patient or client support networks to work on solutions.

We recommend the person-centered emergency planning (P-CEP) concepts and tools. Resources and tools can be obtained from Collaborating4Inclusion (https://collaborating4inclus ion.org/home/pcep/—Resources, Toolkit, Short Course). This person-centered approach to emergency planning has been co-produced and tested in communities including older people and people with disability. Each person's emergency plan will be different, as each person's capabilities and resources are different.

The key principles of person-centered emergency planning are:

1.   **Have the conversation**

The first step is to have the conversation. This is followed by looking at what is already in place, and what is known about emergency risks where you live (and unfortunately Australia is prone to fires, floods, droughts, extreme heat, climate change, and pandemics).

2. **Be as well as possible**

    Now we need to get everyday life and chronic conditions under control. Older people may need to talk to their GP to access referrals and resources, and also to get extra scripts so they can have a supply in their emergency kit.

3. **Create an emergency kit**

    This means having supplies for surviving a week with no food, water, power, medication deliveries: essential medications, first aid kit, bottled water for a week (look for a brand that older hands with reduced dexterity can easily open unaided), large container of disinfectant, emergency food supplies, batteries and a flashlight/torch/portable radio (talk to your GP or social support provider if you won't be able to hear a radio, amplified ear buds or a personal amplifier may be of use here but you will need spare batteries for everything).

    Each person's emergency kit will be different as each person's capabilities and resources are different. Don't forget pet food supplies and to check every year that the contents of your kit are still "in date" and safe to consume.

4. **Establish and maintain social connections**

    Informal supports are critical in an emergency: This means communicating with family, friends, support workers, and community organizations. This also means knowing who neighbors are even if it is just for a brief conversation. Knowing what support people can and can't offer in an emergency is important.

5. **Communicate the plan**

    Finally, the plan should be communicated to everyone in your support network, so everyone knows. If there are gaps or missing supports, everyone should collaborate to find a solution or alternatives.

A real life example

Author One shares their emergency plan:

My main need is for communication and given both the hearing loss and low vision, I am sometimes going to need a real person to help me. The principal emergency threat I face is from Covid-19 and my own heightened risk of falls not seeing or hearing enough to safely mobilize all the time.

My key strength is that I am organized!

So, I have a Covid plan so that support workers and family know to COVID test when: 1. Unwell; 2. They come into contact with others who become Covid positive; and 3. Before coming to work. The Covid plan was in force during the last two lockdowns and during November/December 2023 in the middle of an eighth Covid wave (Sydney). I provide RAT tests packets to each worker and replace as needed.

If positive, workers stay away for ten days. If I were to be positive, I don't have anyone come to work for ten days. The GP gives me antivirals and the family provide on-site support. We always have prepared meals in the freezer for emergencies if no one is able to be at home with me.

We have emergency supplies of food, water, medications, anti-bacterial hand wash, wipes, and antiseptic surface sprays stored in the bottom of the pantry.

We use the haptic emergency signal of a cross on the back for anyone in my network to alert me to the need to follow now and ask questions later.

We use text messages to communicate between my support network and family. Key supports are on speed dial. It is also well known that if I make a phone call, then it is an emergency, and they are to come and help or send help in the form of an ambulance. This has been one of the great fears that I am not able to arrange and manage a call to emergency services myself.

Health information is in the health app on my smartphone as well as in the hospital preparedness kit on my bedroom door. This contains a "deafblind" wristband, tactile communication resources (social-haptics communication, deafblind manual alphabet chart, and tactile signs for emergencies and hospital use). See earlier section on going to hospital.

A fire blanket and a fire extinguisher are in the laundry, as when we had a gas cooktop I set fire to myself and a kitchen cupboard accidentally. As a safety precaution, we recently switched to an induction cooktop. A second fire extinguisher sits in the foyer.

I also have a smart watch, which contains a fall detector that will activate an ambulance call if I don't click that I am okay after a fall.

Just because I have DSI doesn't mean that I am not responsible for the care of other people. I have a 95-year-old neighbor and we look out for each other. In an emergency, I will look out for her as well as myself and vice versa. I have a partner and family, and I need to be able to get help for them if necessary, too. This is why my network needs to extend beyond just my partner and immediate family.

The plan has been communicated widely as for example the emergency social-haptic signal is of no use if no one else knows it. As the need arises, we check and change aspects of the plan and the physical and social supports we might need. The plan is documented and held in the support worker handbook as well as the training each receives; family members know their roles and responsibilities, as do I. We haven't yet "solved" the issue of communication during an emergency but at present, the use of text messages (in an accessible way with dark mode and large font) is working. Because this is so critical, we have included power banks in our emergency kit (that are recharged periodically) so that a power reserve is available in a power outage situation.

Conclusion

Being prepared is critical to saving lives, maintaining independence, and minimizing negative experiences. We, as health and social care students, professionals, as carers families and friends, as support networks, and as people living with complexities and sensory impairments need to collaborate to get our figurative ducks in a row, actively plan, and prepare for the next hospitalization and the next emergency.

11
Living better with DSI

Integration of care: Putting it all together

How it all works together

We present Lucy's story as an illustration of how integration of care can work. Using verbatim testimony we can walk through Lucy's dual sensory impairment (DSI) journey. Lucy is 80 years of age, lives in outer suburban Sydney, and tells how the combination of sensory losses and the death of her main communication partner, her husband Walter, had significant social, health, and wellbeing consequences. It is not uncommon for older people to experience a crisis following the loss of a key support (Dunsmore, 2022). With the loss of Walter, Lucy gave up a beloved hobby, bridge playing, as well as isolating herself from church, interests, and friends.

To recap earlier chapters–DSI is common and impacts more women as they tend to live longer. The Australian data tell us:

- 66% of people over 60 years have hearing loss (House of Representative Standing Committee on Health, Aged Care and Sport 2017)

- 6.5% of those 50 years or older have visual impairment (Foreman et al., 2017)
- Both of these increase with age until more than one in four have DSI at age 80 (Schneider et al., 2012)

And for those older people living with DSI, life becomes complicated, with increased risk of:

- Difficulty with activities of daily living and instrumental activities (Brennan et al., 2005; Brennan et al., 2006; Guthrie et al., 2018)
- Cognitive decline (Davidson & Guthrie, 2019; Lin et al., 2004; Tay et al., 2006)
- Dementia (Kuo et al., 2021)
- Communication breakdowns (Heine and Browning, 2002, 2004)
- Decreased social participation, fewer contacts (Crews and Campbell, 2004; Dunsmore, 2022; Jaiswal et al., 2020; Lind et al., 2003; Mick et al., 2018; Viljanin et al., 2013)
- Reduced wellbeing, increased depression (Capella-McDonnall, 2005; 2009; Harada et al., 2008; Kiely et al., 2013; Lehane et al., 2018)
- Reduced quality of life (Chia et al., 2006; Tseng et al., 2018)
- Increased mortality risk (Gopinath et al., 2013; Zhang et al., 2020)
- Increased likelihood of delirium (Cacchione et al., 2003)
- Visual hallucinations (Vukicevic and Fitzmaurice, 2008; Pang, 2016)
- Other complications can involve falls risk, decreased public messaging awareness, poorer healthcare experiences (Watharow, 2023).

Reported negative impacts provide a picture of troubling associations for those with DSI, (see earlier chapters for more detail). Most of the studies referred to are quantitative studies, so they don't authentically convey what it's like to be an older person with DSI, where one sense cannot compensate for the other. There are potential and real difficulties in all social domains especially around communication, access to information, and orientation and mobility. This means that for those with DSI, information is received in unreliable fragments, physical environments can be hazardous, and social encounters are fraught.

To put a personal lived experience perspective to this invisible epidemic, Lucy tells us what DSI is like for her. We will explore what happened in the absence of a dedicated diagnostic or support service. And how that changed as Lucy, and her super team of friends, carers, family, GP, community nursing team, ophthalmologist, audiologist, exercise physiologist, tactile teacher, and others, all acquired useful skills. There is reciprocity in sharing insights and learning with each other. Since we don't yet have a dedicated service that is fully funded to support older Australians living with DSI and their families/carers, this mutual learning is critical.

Lucy says:

> It's been very difficult since Walter died, as you know, and then the Covid. I'm so wobbly now. Bit scared to leave the house in case I fall. Lot scared really. Barry's in Perth, and so no use to me, but his eldest, my granddaughter, Natalie, is moving to Sydney to do Uni here. I hope she'll visit…it's been hard. Too hard keeping up with my

friends and because they can't understand. I can't walk into a room. I see nothing and I can't find my seat and I can't recognize people. It's really hard to listen. No, not hard to listen but to hear. I try to work it out, but none of it makes any sense, you see. I know it's just old age, but I'm finding it all difficult. I do feel bad when everyone has invited me out to their houses, but I can't invite them back because it's too tricky to make a cup of tea. I worry I might scald myself. And I do burn myself making biscuits. So, I've stopped all that cooking. And bridge! I loved bridge. We weren't often beaten, Walter and I, but when I went on my own, I started to offend people because they don't know about the bad ears and eyes. I look the same I take it, and they forget. Everyone forgets. You might have told them, but they forget…naturally…and the women that I have known at the club for years—well I find that I wouldn't recognize them. I know what they're thinking. She's snobby now. They've all forgotten. You see they've forgotten that I am not able to see them. So, I finally thought, I'll give it away. But once you give it away you lose contact. I keep away from people. I'm all right one to one, but I don't like going out anymore because I can't keep in the conversation. I can't hear it. (for access to the video vignette of Lucy's Story email Author One)

Discussion

Lucy is clearly describing difficulties with anxiety, fear of falls, of burns and scalds, accidents, the misconceptions of others, difficulty understanding what is being said, and increasing social isolation. So, how did Lucy get help?

The family asked Lucy's GP and family practice registered nurse for help. Lucy had commented that the practice team were usually too busy with all her other illnesses such as high blood pressure and diabetes to address her "not seeing too well or hearing too good." So, Lucy's family made a specific appointment to discuss the struggles with daily life and her social withdrawal with her GP and practice nurse. The good news was the GP said we can do things to help, firstly, let's get diagnosed.

A hearing health check showed severe presbycusis (age related hearing loss). An ophthalmologic review confirmed age-related macular degeneration. So, the audiologist was able to certify Lucy as a complex case, which meant the government provided higher subsidies for assistive devices such as hearing aids, doorbell ringers, flashing/vibrating smoke alarms, vibrating alarm clocks etc. The ophthalmologist referred Lucy to Vision Australian (a disability organization supporting those with low vision) for general support including orientation and mobility training. Lucy now had the beginnings of a super team managed and coordinated by the GP and practice nurse. A social worker with counselling skills and experience with older people also became involved. The GP is a colleague of Author One and asked for more information and advice. They noted, "There is not much out there (on DSI)."

We asked Lucy what **she** wanted from life. Lucy replied that she wanted her life back from before, "with the bridge club, the church ladies and my family." The GP wanted Lucy to be in better physical shape and self-managing her other conditions. The family wanted her to be happier.

We suggested starting with communication basics as Lucy needed to understand what everyone was saying so she would be able to contribute actively, rather than saying "yes" to everything without comprehending the substance of the conversation. Lucy now has a notebook in her handbag and another on the coffee table. She also has a thick black pen for use with these.

Visits with the audiologist

Two hearing aids were fitted but Lucy found they made some sounds much worse (e.g., ambient noise in group settings) and she had headaches after wearing them. Furthermore, the aids were not providing enough amplification and clarity to follow television shows or conversations. After five months, the hearing aids were not consistently being worn and spent most of the week in the bedside table drawer. It was obvious that everyone involved needed to accept that this wasn't solving any of Lucy's issues and had in fact become another one. The audiologist suggested that using a personal amplifier for important conversations might be the best bet and to just let Lucy navigate her sensory loss with other methods.

Practical supports

Natalie, Lucy's granddaughter set her up with customizable subtitles on the TV (large font, yellow on black worked best for Lucy). The local library added Lucy to the home delivery library service of large print titles which pleased Lucy. No one had much success teaching apps and accessibility features on a smart phone to Lucy, so this was set aside. Lucy's son bought her an iPad for Christmas, and this was more successful due to the size of the icons and buttons. Lucy now also had an electronic book app that is supported by the local library so she can read large font, dark mode, in yellow print. This pleased Lucy as she loves her mysteries and historical romances.

Cups of tea

A visit to the local low vision support organization and shop was fruitful. On the advice of the occupational therapist, Lucy bought a hot water dispenser. This device allowed her to place her mug under a recessed spout, push a button and one mug of hot water, no more, is dispensed reducing the risk of scalds. Lucy could make her own mugs of tea again, including cups for visitors. She also obtained thick, no bleed, felt tipped pens to use for writing notes, and for others to use to write to her. Some magnifiers were also bought. One of the problems Lucy reports is that she keeps losing everything because she can't always *see* where she has put an item, or if someone else has moved it. So, she says the magnifiers haven't been as useful as they could be if she could reliably find them. They however help with labels on food and use by dates. The occupational therapist suggested she keep one in the kitchen drawer, so it was easily found and replaced.

Transitions

Lucy transitioned to tactile messaging as she needed communication support to augment her residual hearing and vision once hearing aids were officially abandoned. Making a transition to tactile messaging is not confined to those not using hearing aids. Author One uses hearing aids, tactile messaging, tactile sign language, and a manual alphabet for fingerspelling; everyone with DSI needs an individualized collection of what works well and what helps in different situations There are very low levels of awareness amongst medical practitioners and health care practitioners generally, and GPs specifically, about DSI and its myriad complexities.

An important prelude to transitioning to touch based messaging is to establish safe places for others to touch. The sign and haptics teacher who formed part of the super team explored this with Lucy. Lucy didn't want people touching her face, but was happy for tactile messaging on her arms, hands, shoulders, and back.

Documenting strategies

We advised (strongly) that a communication book be started in which all the signs, messages, and strategies would be written out and described. We believe it is imperative that all communication assistive strategies need to be documented so that others (e.g., family, friends, GPs, health and social care professionals, support workers etc.) can access the methods in use. This helps with pivoting from one method to another, as well as focusing on improving communication with a good understanding of what might be needed. Most with DSI will experience changes as their conditions may progress. This means new methods and signs may be needed in time. The book then is a record of everything that is in use.

Emergency sign

It is important that learning tactile messaging takes place with a communication partner (how can anyone practice without one?) Natalie, Lucy's granddaughter, joins her for most sessions. They begin with the tactile sign for an emergency: The cross on the back which means come with me and don't talk or delay, I will explain later. Indeed, Natalie used her finger to outline a large X on her grandmother's back when there was a gas leak in a building they were in. An emergency evacuation order was given over a loudspeaker. Lucy had no idea what was being said. This emergency highlighted the utility of a touch-based emergency message. It was explained to everyone that this was a serious sign and that it was not to be used in non-emergencies.

Fingerspelling

We followed this with the deafblind manual alphabet. Natalie, the granddaughter, learned this very quickly, but Lucy needed several weeks. She also needed large print pictures as shown in chapters 8 and 9. Next, the teacher introduced the friends from church to the manual alphabet and fingerspelling which helped Lucy's church friends recall Lucy's DSI. We are all learning that older adults with DSI take longer to learn the manual alphabet than younger people and need lots of different ways to absorb the material. Many games were played such as, "I went shopping and I bought…" and finger spelling was practiced using the manual alphabet to spell out items such as tea, bread, chocolate, apples.

The church ladies

Lucy also learned to put her hand out as a signal to her communication partners that she needed a topic or sentence tactilely communicated to her. The church ladies came religiously once a week, and talked about how useful this could be for other people they know, underscoring how sensory loss is common in older people. These ladies know of others in their communities who were struggling with sensory loss or losses and felt better able to understand and remember what their friends were going through. This is a timely reminder of how common, yet invisible, sensory loss in older people is.

Risk factors become reality

Progress was interrupted when Lucy had a fall in the bathroom and broke her upper arm. She had been on a wait list for an occupational therapy assessment of her home environment. During this hospitalization Lucy developed vivid visual hallucinations. She told Natalie, "I think I have the dementia." Lucy was not given any communication support during her stay, and in fact did not know she needed to have another surgery in the future. There was some confusion after discharge as Lucy was unsure what medications she should take as she had neither heard what the doctor/nurse said and there were no large print instructions. It was a long weekend, so her GP surgery was closed. This reinforced to Lucy, her family, and GP, that formal discharge planning would be a must in any future hospital admission. The GP and the ophthalmologist reassured Lucy her hallucinations were related to the stress of the accident and surgery and not a sign of something sinister like dementia. Lucy, over time, became less troubled by these.

Health haptics and super teams

Following this unwelcome interruption, Lucy began to learn some health haptics, adding them to the communication book.

The GP and practice nurse team also helped Natalie and Lucy begin gathering everything they would need for a going to hospital kit. A photocopy of the communication book was included as was a laminated card displaying the large-print manual alphabet for fingerspelling, haptics, and other touch messaging methods. There are electronic versions for those with devices, digital know-how, and sufficient residual vision. Generally, for older adults with acquired low vision, use of technology is lower than for younger age groups. Natalie added a new notebook and several thick textas. This has all been put in a bright yellow cloth bag that lives on the hall table in case it is needed.

Some examples of the health haptics used:

- Needle and where on the body
- Hurting and where on the body
- Doctor /nurse
- Be still
- Okay?
- Take tablets
- Blood pressure check and other observations (see Chapter 8 for images and full descriptions)

Lucy and her practice nurse were able to use the health haptics for a "needle" in the upper arm when she received a set of vaccinations ahead of the winter influenza season. The GP arranged for an aged care assessment team to review Lucy and they organized support hours at home. So now Lucy has one hour a day, five days a week. Natalie comes to assist on weekends but for many older people with DSI, there are hours, days, weekends, and weeks without adequate social care.

Short cuts

Lucy, Natalie, and the church friends also learned a few short cuts: based on Auslan tactile sign language. These included:

- Yes and No
- Tea
- Coffee
- Shopping
- Laughing
- Crying/sad

These are done on Lucy's palm. Yes and No signs can also be done on the upper arm. When Lucy is talking to her friends, whoever is sitting next to her can make the Yes sign on her upper arm to indicate people are agreeing with her. When people are laughing, her companion can signal this by a round handshape on the upper arm with the fingers moving rapidly. We all can forget that this sort of feedback is important in social settings.

Guiding haptics

Social haptics was next, a little out of order than was initially planned owing to the emergency hospital admission. These adaptable touch messages on the upper arm, hand or back included:

- Identifying who is in the room or more importantly at the bridge table.
- Sighted guiding: stop, stairs, escalators, down, up, uneven terrain.

Bridge again?

The next step was to help Lucy (re)build happier social connections starting now with bridge haptics. Bridge was very important to Lucy in the past and its loss was the source of much grief. The bridge club agreed to use large print cards for everyone (and this actually helped quite a few other players feel more comfortable). This is a valuable example of an accommodation for one that helps others too. Lucy learned touch signals for the different bids and one of the church ladies who also played bridge but for a different group went along as Lucy's support for several sessions to help facilitate and teach the new touch messages for bids and tricks. This was more complicated because there was some resistance by other players who suspected touch messaging could be used to cheat. This proved to be insurmountable as several club members refused to play with Lucy.

Travel

Lucy's son lives five hours by plane away and a trip to visit was booked. Natalie would accompany Lucy, but Lucy would need specific strategies to manage the trip. Visual signifiers for staff were also suggested here and Lucy wore a lanyard which had deafblind on it in very large letters. Some travel touch messages Lucy used included: Stop, put your hands out (for hand swabs), and another for Star position for some of the body scanners. This was in addition to liaising for assistance via the airline. Her son had a training session by Zoom before her arrival and Natalie could help her father and her grandmother communicate and practice. Natalie said there was a lot of laughter over some of the fingerspelling mistakes because her father's spelling was not the best. He kept getting his B's and G's mixed up, bun became gun, for example.

Physical health

Lucy had been deconditioned by her social and physical withdrawal and social isolation at home for so long. One key goal the GP had was to get her moving again. They explained that this would help her diabetes and bone health as well as general wellbeing. The GP made a referral to an exercise physiologist. The exercise physiologist came to Lucy's house and quickly understood that touch messaging on the shoulder and upper arm would help them communicate with Lucy.

These messages included:

- That's right/you are doing well
- Turn around
- Sit to stand
- Kickbacks/sidekicks
- Heel raises

With the co-creation of touch messages, Lucy was able to engage in her supervised program. The exercise physiologist also devised a plan for unsupervised activities such as chair exercises with kickouts/arm raises and sit to stands. Natalie took walks with Lucy when she visited using the guiding haptics with messages for stop/turn around/step up/step down. Rough or uneven ground ahead was signaled with Natalie's hand on Lucy's hand (which is in the crook of her elbow), the fingers moving up and down randomly to signify uneven terrain.

Name signs

It was important to have name signs to explain who was in the room, who as coming and going, and where people were sitting. The name signs had to be ones that Lucy understood and so her contribution and approval was needed for each. Everyone had a lot of fun with this one and they used a mixture of manual alphabet, drawings and actions on the upper arm or hand and were very individual with idiosyncrasies representing the diversity of humans. Some examples where:

- Natalie: Two fingers on the upper arm (representing N for Natalie with the fingers trailing down the arm signifying her very long hair)
- Walter: Lucy's husband had a sign because he was often referred to conversation this name sign was a double tap to Lucy's wedding ring

We don't want you to think this was an overnight success or that everything occurred in linear fashion. It wasn't. And it didn't. The GP had to construct a super team from their own connections (and involvement with the authors) as no stand-alone national DSI comprehensive and integrated support service exists where Lucy lives.

While Lucy's granddaughter learned quickly, everyone else took many months to work out what signs were useful and what weren't and then to remember them. Lucy is a slow finger speller, so no one needs to be fast. Natalie has to remember to slow down. These measures do not replace language but provide ways to augment communication with short messages and contextual information. This reduces communication tension and frustration. What we have all learned is that repetition and revision, pivoting and co-producing new signals are ongoing processes. And our experiences highlight the burning need for Federal government recognition, funding, and establishment of integrated DSI services.

Social wins (and exits)

If Lucy went out, social haptics' skills meant that her companion could indicate on her back where everyone was sitting by drawing a rectangle first, then pressing with one finger to give the location of Lucy, as everyone else will be relative to that orientation. Using the name signs or fingerspelling or spoken names if Lucy can hear them, means Lucy can know where everyone is sitting. This is useful in restaurants or gatherings over a meal or church morning teas. As Lucy started going out more there were setbacks when she felt she just couldn't cope. She noted, "I need a get-me-out-of-here sign." This sign works in reverse, Lucy can draw a small cross on her companion's hand that means "I'm not coping. Do something." That something may be to explain to Lucy what is happening or to collect their things, say goodbye, and leave the event. But, it gives Lucy some control over difficult social situations.

Resources

Everyone needed tangible resources to practice and review the various tactile messaging methods. We shared laminated cards of the various systems from the communication book. This meant there was a dictionary of sorts that is specific for Lucy and her particular social network. It is also a resource for the various carers that have been coming in for an hour a day during the week as part of her aged care package. There is high turnover of carers, so the support workers are not always completely *au fait* with Lucy's tactile messaging but the tension around communication and Lucy's social isolation have both been reduced. One support worker commented that they were worried they would never learn all the alphabet and signs and be too slow. Then they realised that they didn't have to be fast because Lucy couldn't keep up. "This is slow conversation."

BDBD

BDBD is short for bad deafblind day and one of Author One's friends coined it to inject a bit of humor into times when eyes and ears just don't work well at anything. Fatigue, stress, or a busy few days can mean any day can become a BDBD (or a BDSID). Sometimes Lucy isn't really across any of the methods especially as she says, "as my eyes get worse, I get deafer too." One coping mechanism has been that Lucy asks questions and Natalie or a friend reply with Yes or No on her arm or palm. Some days that's more than enough.

These methods and measures aren't a prescription for everyone. In the absence of dedicated services and policies in Australia, Lucy's journey with DSI was very much *ad hoc* and iterative. A super team evolved that took stock every six months with Lucy and the GP, and annually with Lucy and the ophthalmologist. The ophthalmologist noted that they had a better grasp of DSI that informed their practice going forwards. This was a direct result of increased awareness from being involved in the super team. Each individual and each family living with DSI will be different.

The important thing is to respond to individual goals and needs as not only does each person's vary but also because goals and needs may vary over time.

Conclusion

There is an invisible epidemic among older people of single and dual sensory impairment. As our populations rapidly age, live longer, and with more impairments and conditions, more are at risk of unseen, unheard DSI. Our purpose in writing this book is fourfold: 1. Campaign for distinct disability status for deafblindness/dual sensory impairment; 2. Highlight the need for policymakers to recognize and address these pressing issues in health care, communication, and social life for older people with DSI; 3. To address the education of our future health and social care providers by raising awareness of DSI in older people; 4. Finally, to show that social isolation, communication tension, and exile from the things we love doing can be mitigated. Older people with DSI can live happier, healthier, safer lives.

Bibliography

Abley, C., Bond, J., and Robinson, L. (2011). Improving Interprofessional Practice for Vulnerable Older People: Gaining a Better Understanding of Vulnerability. *Journal of Interprofessional Care*, 25(5), pp. 359–365. https://doi.org/10.3109/13561 820.2011.579195

Urqueta Alfaro, A., McGraw, C., Guthrie, D. M. and Wittich, W. (2021). Optimizing Evaluation of Older Adults with Vision and/or Hearing Loss Using the interRAI Community Health Assessment and Deafblind Supplement. *Frontiers in Rehabilitation Sciences*, 2, 764022.

Amare, A. T., Caughey, G. E., Whitehead, C., Lang, C. E., Bray, S. C., Corlis, M., Visvanathan, R., Wesselingh, S. and Inacio, M. C. (2020). The Prevalence, Trends and Determinants of Mental Health Disorders in Older Australians Living in Permanent Residential Aged Care: Implications for Policy and Quality of Aged Care Services. *Australian & New Zealand Journal of Psychiatry*, 54(12), pp. 1200–1211. https://doi.org/10.1177/0004867420945367

Andrews, E. E., Ayers, K. B., Brown, K. S., Dunn, D. S. and Pilarski, C. R. (2021). No Body Is Expendable: Medical Rationing and Disability Justice During the COVID-19 Pandemic. *American Psychologist*, 76(3), pp. 451–461. https://doi.org/10.1037/amp0000709

Antonelli, M. T., Grace, P. J. and Boltz, M. (2020). Mutual Caregiving: Living Meaningfully as an Older Couple. *International Journal of Older People Nursing*, 15(4), Article e12340. https://doi.org/10.1111/opn.12340

Antonucci, T. C. (2001). Social relations: An examination of social networks, social support, and sense of control. In: J. E. Birren and K. W. Schaie, eds., *Handbook of the Psychology of Ageing*. Academic Press, pp. 427–453

Antonucci, T. C., Ajrouch, K. J. and Birditt, K. S. (2014). The Convoy Model: Explaining Social Relations From a Multidisciplinary Perspective. *The Gerontologist*, 54(1), pp. 82–92. https://doi.org/10.1093/geront/gnt118

Australian Bureau of Statistics. (2018). *Disability, ageing and carers, Australia: Summary of findings*. [Online] Available at: www.abs.gov.au/statistics/health/disability/disability-ageing-and-carers-australia-summary-findings/latest-release

Australian Bureau of Statistics. (2019). *Disability, aging and carers, summary of findings*. https://www.aihw.gov.au/reports/australias-disability-strategy/australias-disability-strategy-outcomes-framework/contents/about

Australian Bureau of Statistics. (2020). *Twenty years of population change*. https://www.abs.gov.au/articles/twenty-years-population-change

Australian Government Department of Health. (2020). *Types of aged care: Care in your home*. [Online] Available at: www.health.gov.au/health-topics/aged-care/about-aged-care/types-of-aged-care#care-in-your-home

Australian Government, House of Representatives Standing Committee on Health, aged care and Sport. (2017) *Still waiting to be heard … Report on the Inquiry into the Hearing Health and Wellbeing of Australia*. [Online] Available at: https://parlinfo.aph.gov.au/parlInfo/download/committees/reportrep/024048/toc_pdf/Stillwaitingtobeheard….pdf;fileType=application/pdf.

Australian Government. (n.d.). *My aged care: Commonwealth Home Support Programme*. [Online] Available at: www.myagedcare.gov.au/help-at-home/commonwealth-home-support-programme

Australian Government. (2021a). *Royal Commission into Aged Care Quality and Safety – Final report: A summary of the final report*. https://agedcare.royalcommission.gov.au/publications/final-report

Australian Government. (2021b). *Royal Commission into Aged Care Quality and Safety – Final report: List of recommendations*. https://agedcare.royalcommission.gov.au/publications/final-report

Australian Government. (2022). *My Aged Care: Home care packages*. https://www.myagedcare.gov.au/help-at-home/home-care-packages

Australian Human Rights Commission. (2013). *Fact or fiction? Stereotypes of older Australians: Research report 2013*. https://humanrights.gov.au/our-work/age-discrimination/publications/fact-or-fiction-stereotypes-older-australians-research

Australian Institute of Health and Welfare. (2019). *Homelessness and homelessness services*. [Online] Available at: www.aihw.gov.au/reports/australias-welfare/homelessness-and-homelessness-services

Australian Institute of Health and Welfare. (2020, July 23). *Australia's health: Indigenous health*. [Online] Available at: www.aihw.gov.au/reports/australias-health/indigenous-hearing-health

Avery, S. (2020). Aboriginal and Torres Strait Islander People with Disability: Falling Through the Cracks. *PRECEDENT*, 159, pp. 12–15.

Avery, S. (2018). *Culture is inclusion: A narrative of Aboriginal and Torres Strait Islander people with disability*.

Ayalon, L., & Tesch-Römer, C. (2017). Taking a closer look at ageism: Self- and other-directed ageist attitudes and discrimination. *European Journal of Ageing, 14*(1), pp. 1–4. https://doi.org/10.1007/s10433-016-0409-9

Badr, H., Carmack, C. L., Kashy, D. A., Cristofanilli, M. and Revenson, T. A. (2010). Dyadic Coping in Metastatic Breast Cancer. *Health Psychology*, 29(2), pp. 169–180. https://doi.org/10.1037/a0018165

Baguley, D., McFerran, D. and Hall, D. (2013) Tinnitus. *Lancet*, 382, pp. 1600–1607.

Barker, A. B., Leighton, P. and Ferguson, M. A. (2017). Coping Together with Hearing Loss: A Qualitative Meta-synthesis of the Psychosocial Experiences of People with Hearing Loss and their Communication partners. *International Journal of Audiology*, 56(5), pp. 297–305. https://doi.org/10.1080/14992027.2017.1286695

Barnes, M. (2015). Beyond the dyad: Exploring the multidimensionality of care in Tula Brannelly, Lizzie Ward, and Nicki Ward (eds), *Ethics of Care: Critical advances in international perspective* (Bristol, 2015; online edn, Policy Press Scholarship Online, 19 May 2016), https://doi.org/10.1332/policypress/9781447316510.003.0003, accessed 11 June 2024.

Bartlett, G., Blaid, R., Tamblyn, R., Clermont, R. J. and MacGibbon, B. (2008). Impact of Patient Communication Problems on the Risk of Preventable Adverse Events in Acute Care Settings. *Canadian Medical Association Journal*, 178(12), pp. 1555–1562. https://doi.org/10.1503/cmaj.070690

Bauer, C. A. (2018). Tinnitus. *New English Journal of Medicine*. Mar 29; 378(13), pp. 1224-1231. https://doi.org/10.1056/NEJMcp1506631

Beard, J. R., Officer, A., de Carvalho, I. A., Sadana, R., Pot, A. M., Michel, J. P., Lloyd-Sherlock, P., Epping-Jordan, J. E., Peeters, G., Mahanani, W. R., Thiyagarajan, J. A. and Chatterji, S. (2016). The World Report on Ageing and Health: A Policy Framework for Healthy Ageing. *The Lancet*, 387(10033), pp. 2145–2154. https://doi.org/10.1016/S0140-6736(15)00516-4

Berg, C. A. and Upchurch, R. (2007). A Developmental-Contextual Model of Couples Coping with Chronic Illness Across the Adult Life Span. *Psychological Bulletin*, 133(6), pp. 920–954. https://doi.org/10.1037/0033-2909.133.6.920

Berghs, M., Atkin, K., Graham, H., Hatton, C. and Thomas, C. (2016). Implications for Public Health Research of Models and Theories of Disability: A Scoping Study and Evidence Synthesis. *Public Health Research*, 4(8). https://doi.org/10.3310/phr04080

Berkman, L. F., Glass, T., Brissette, I. and Seeman, T. E. (2000). From Social Integration to Health: Durkheim in the New Millennium. *Social Science & Medicine*, 51(6), pp. 843–857. https://doi.org/10.1016/s0277-9536(00)00065-4

Berkman, L. F. and Syme, S. L. (1979). Social Networks, Host Resistance, and Mortality: A Nine-Year Follow-Up Study of Alameda County Residents. *American Journal of Epidemiology*, 109(2), pp. 186–204. https://doi.org/10.1093/oxfordjournals.aje.a112674

Bertschi, I. C., Meier, F. and Bodenmann, G. (2021). Disability as an Interpersonal Experience: A Systematic Review on Dyadic Challenges and Dyadic Coping When One Partner has a Chronic Physical or Sensory Impairment. *Frontiers in Psychology*, 12, Article 624609. https://doi.org/10.3389/fpsyg.2021.624609

Beukes, E. W., Ulep, A. J., Andersson, G. and Manchaiah, V. (2022) The Effects of Tinnitus on Significant Others. J. Clin. Med. 11, p. 1393. https://doi.org/10.3390/jcm11051393

Beukes, E. W., Andersson, G., & Manchaiah, V. (2023). Third-Party Disability for Significant Others of Individuals with Tinnitus: A Cross-Sectional Survey Design. *Audiology Research (Pavia, Italy)*, *13*(3), 378–388. https://doi.org/10.3390/audiolres13030033

Blair, J. (2019). Diagnostic overshadowing: See beyond the diagnosis. University of Hertfordshire – Intellectual Disability and Health. [Online] Available at: www.intellectualdisability.info/changing-values/diagnostic-overshadowing-see-beyond-the-diagnosis

BMJ 2023. Hearing aids and dementia risk … and other stories. (2023). *BMJ (Online)*, *380*, p135-. https://doi.org/10.1136/bmj.p135

Bodenmann, G. (1997). The influence of stress and coping on close relationships: A two-year longitudinal study. *Swiss Journal of Psychology*, *56*(3), 156–164.

Bodenmann, G. (2005). Dyadic coping and its significance for marital functioning. In T. Revenson, K. Kayser, & G. Bodenmann (Eds.), *Couples coping with stress: Emerging perspectives on dyadic coping* (pp. 33–50). American Psychological Association.

Bodsworth, S. M., Clare, I. C. H. and Simblett, S. K. (2011). Deafblindness and Mental Health: Psychological Distress and Unmet Need Among Adults with Dual Sensory Impairment. *British Journal of Visual Impairment*, 29(1), pp. 6–26. https://doi.org/10.1177/0264619610387495

Boisvert, I., Ferguson, M., van Wieringen, A., & Ricketts, T. A. (2022). Outcome Measures to Assess the Benefit of Interventions for Adults with Hearing Loss: From Research to Clinical Application. *Frontiers in Neuroscience*, 16, 955189.

Braun, M., Scholz, U., Bailey, B., Perren, S., Hornung, R. and Martin, M. (2009). Dementia Caregiving in Spousal Relationships: A Dyadic Perspective. *Aging and Mental Health*, 13(3), pp. 426–436. https://doi.org/10.1080/13607860902879441

Brennan, M. and Bally, S. J. (2007). Psychosocial Adaptations to Dual Sensory Loss in Middle and Late Adulthood. *Trends in Amplification*, 11(4), pp. 281–300. https://doi.org/10.1177/10847 13807308210

Brennan, M., Horowitz, A. and Su, Y.-P. (2005). Dual Sensory Loss and its Impact on Everyday Competence. *The Gerontologist*, 45(3), pp. 337–346. https://doi.org/10.1093/geront/45.3.337

Bucholc, M., McClean, P. L., Bauermeister, S., Todd, S., Ding, X., Ye, Q., … and Maguire, L. P. (2021). Association of the Use of Hearing Aids with the Conversion from Mild Cognitive Impairment to Dementia and Progression of Dementia: A Longitudinal Retrospective Study. *Alzheimer's & Dementia: Translational Research & Clinical Interventions*, 7(1), e12122. https://doi.org/10.1002/trc2.12122

Burton, A. E., Shaw, R. L. and Gibson, J. M. (2015). Living Together with Age-Related Macular Degeneration: An Interpretative Phenomenological Analysis of Sense-Making Within a Dyadic Relationship. *Journal of Health Psychology*, 20(10), pp. 1285–1295. https://doi.org/10.1177/1359105313511134

Burri, A., Blank Gebre, M., & Bodenmann, G. (2017). Individual and dyadic coping in chronic pain patients. *Journal of Pain Research*, 10, pp. 535–544. https://doi.org/10.2147/JPR.S128871

Buyukgol, H., Gunes, E. and Eren, F. A. (2018). Alice in Wonderland Syndrome: A Case Report. *J. Neurosci. Neuropsychol*, 2, p. 101.

Cacchione, P. Z., Culp, K., Dyck, M. J. and Laing, J. (2003). Risk for Acute Confusion in Sensory-Impaired, Rural, Long-Term-Care Elders. *Clinical Nursing Research*, 12(4), pp. 340–355.

Cacioppo, J. T. and Cacioppo, S. (2014). Social Relationships and Health: The Toxic Effects of Perceived Social Isolation. *Social and Personality Psychology Compass*, 8(2), pp. 58–72. https://doi.org/10.1111/spc3.12087

Cacioppo, J. T., Hawkley, L. C., Crawford, L. E., Ernst, J. M., Burleson, M. H., Kowalewski, R. B., Malarkey, W. B., Van Cauter, E., & Berntson, G. G. (2002). Loneliness and health: Potential mechanisms, *Psychosomatic Medicine*, *64*(3), 407–417. https://doi.org/10.1097/00006842-200205000-00005

Calgaro, E., Craig, N., Craig, L., Dominey-Howes, D. and Allen, J. (2021). Silent no More: Identifying and Breaking Through the Barriers that d/Deaf People Face in Responding to Hazards and Disasters. *International Journal of Disaster Risk Reduction*, 57. https://doi.org/10.1016/j.ijdrr.2021.102156

Cantin, S., Duquette, J., Dutrisac, F., Ponton, L.., Courchesne, M., de Abreu Cybis, W., Montisci, K., Wittich, W., and Wanet-Defalque, M. C. (2019). 'Charles Bonnet syndrome: development and validation of a screening and multidimensional descriptive questionnaire', *Canadian journal of ophthalmology*, 54(3), pp. 323–327.

Carpenter, B. D. and Mak, W. (2007). Caregiving Couples. *Generations*, 31(3), pp. 47–53. https://www.jstor.org/stable/26555541

Charles Bonnet Syndrome Foundation. (2023). [Online] Available at: www.charlesbonnetsyndrome.org/index.php/homepage

Choi, J. S., Adams, M. E., Crimmins, E. M., Lin, F. R. and Ailshire, J. A. (2024). Association Between Hearing Aid Use and Mortality in Adults with Hearing Loss in the USA: A Mortality Follow-Up Study of a Cross-Sectional Cohort. *The Lancet Healthy Longevity*, 5(1), pp. 66–75. https://doi.org/10.1016/S2666-7568(23)00265-9

Cleary, M., Freeman, A. and Walter, G. (2006). Carer Participation in Mental Health Service Delivery. *International Journal of Mental Health Nursing*, 15(3), pp. 189–194. https://doi.org/10.1111/j.1447-0349.2006.00422.x

Cloutier-Fisher, D., Kobayashi, K. and Smith, A. (2011). The Subjective Dimensions of Social Isolation: A Qualitative Investigation of Older Adults' Experience in Small Social Support Networks. *Journal of Aging Studies*, 25(4), pp. 407–414. https://doi.org/10.1016/j.jaging.2011.03.012

Commonwealth of Australia, House of Representatives Standing Committee on Health, Aged Care and Sport. (2017). Still waiting to be heard… report on the Inquiry into the Hearing Health and Wellbeing of Australia. Canberra: Commonwealth of Australia; 2017. [Online] Available at: www.aph.gov.au/Parliamentary_B usiness/Committees/House/Health_Aged_Care_and_Sport/ HearingHealth/Report_1

Corker, M. (1998). Postmodern World. *Disability Reader: Social Science Perspectives. London: Continuum*, 221–233.

Cornwell, B. and Schafer, M. H. (2016). Social networks in later life. In: L. K. George and K. F. Ferraro, eds., *Handbook of Aging and the Social Sciences* (8th ed.). Academic Press, pp. 181–201. https://doi. org/10.1016/b978-0-12-417235-7.00009-3

Coulter, A. and Oldham, J. (2016). Person-Centred Care: What Is It and How Do We Get There? *Future Hospital Journal*, 3(2), pp. 114–116. https://doi.org/10.7861/futurehosp.3-2-114

Cox, T. M. and Ffytche, D. H. (2014). Negative Outcome Charles Bonnet Syndrome. *British Journal of Ophthalmology*, 98, pp. 1236–1239.

Cummins R, Hughes J, Tomyn A, Gibson A, Woerner J, Lai L. (2007) The Wellbeing of Australians-Carer Health and Wellbeing. Australian Unity Wellbeing Index Survey 17.1, Deakin University, Carers Australia, Australian Unity. Available from URL: http:// www.deakin.edu.au/research/acqol/auwbi/survey-reports/sur- vey017-1-report.pdf

Cunnett, J. (2010). *What does good look like? A report of a series of focus groups run with patients and patient representatives at Mid Staffordshire NHS Foundation Trust during September 2010*. Patient and Public Involvement Solutions, UK.

Dalby, D. M., Hirdes, J. P., Stolee, P., Strong, J. G., Poss, J., Tjam, E. Y., Bowman, L. and Ashworth, M. (2009). Characteristics of Individuals with Congenital and Acquired Deaf-Blindness. *Journal of Visual Impairment & Blindness*, 103(2), pp. 93–102. https://doi.org/10.1177/0145482X0910300208

Dammeyer, J. (2010). Prevalence and Aetiology of Congenitally Deafblind People in Denmark. *International Journal of Audiology*, 49(2), pp. 76–82.

Dammeyer, J. (2012). Development and Characteristics of Children with Usher Syndrome and CHARGE Syndrome. *International Journal of Pediatric Otorhinolaryngology*, 76(9), pp. 1292–1296.

Dammeyer, J. (2014). Deafblindness: A Review of the Literature. *Scandinavian Journal of Public Health*, 42(7), pp. 554–562. https://doi.org/10.1177/1403494814544399

Das, A., Babu, G. N., Gupta, A., Kanaujia, V. and Paliwal, V. K. (2020). Vivid Visual Hallucinations in Visually Impaired: Charles Bonnet Syndrome – An Analog to "Phantom-Limb Phenomenon". *Annals of Indian Academy of Neurology*, 23(5), pp. 734–735. https://doi.org/10.4103/aian.AIAN_40_20

David, D., Zoizner, G. and Werner, P. (2018). Self-Stigma and Age-Related Hearing Loss: A Qualitative Study of Stigma Formation and Dimensions. *American Journal of Audiology*, 27(1), pp. 126–136. https://doi.org/10.1044/2017_AJA-17-0050

Davidson, J. G. S. and Guthrie, D. M. (2019). Older Adults With a Combination of Vision and Hearing Impairment Experience Higher Rates of Cognitive Impairment, Functional Dependence, and Worse Outcomes Across a Set of Quality Indicators. *Journal of Aging and Health*, 31(1), pp. 85–108. https://doi.org/10.1177/0898264317723407

Davis, A., McMahon, C. M., Pichora-Fuller, K. M., Russ, S., Lin, F., Olusanya, B. O., Chadha, S. and Tremblay, K. L. (2016). Aging and Hearing Health: The Life-Course Approach. *The Gerontologist*, 56(Suppl. 2), pp. S256–S267. https://doi.org/10.1093/geront/gnw033

Deafblind Nordic Cooperation Committee. (n.d.). *Nordic definition of deafblindness*. [Online] Available at: www.fsdb.org/Filer/DBNSK English.pdf

Deafblind Australia. (2016). *Inquiry into the Hearing Health and Wellbeing of Australia* (Submission 69). Parliament of Australia. [Online] Available at: www.aph.gov.au/Parliamentary_Busin ess/Committees/House/Health_Aged_Care_and_Sport/Hearin gHealth

Deloitte Access Economics. (2020). *The value of informal care in 2020* (Report for Carers Australia). [Online] Available at: www2. deloitte.com/au/en/pages/economics/articles/value-of-infor mal-care-2020.html

Doeller, B., Kratochwil, M., Sifari, L., Hirnschall, N. and Findl, O. (2021). Benefit of Psychiatric Evaluation on Anxiety in Patients with Charles Bonnet Syndrome. *BMJ Open Ophthalmology*, 6(1), e000463–e000463.   https://doi.org/10.1136/bmjophth-2020-000463

Dullard, B. and Saunders, G. H. (2016). Documentation of Dual Sensory Impairment in Electronic Medical Records. *The Gerontologist*, 56(2), pp. 313–317. https://doi.org/10.1093/ger ont/gnu032

Dunsmore, M. E. (2022). *An invisible disability: Navigating the enduring state of dual sensory impairment (DSI) in older age.* PhD thesis, Faculty of Medicine and Health, The University of Sydney, Sydney, Australia.

Dunsmore, M. E., Schneider, J., McKenzie, H. and Gillespie, J. A. (2020). The Effort of Caring: The Caregivers' Perspective of Dual Sensory Impairment. *Frontiers in Education*, 5, Article 572201. https://doi.org/10.3389/feduc.2020.572201

Durai, M., O'Keeffe, M. G. and Searchfield, G. D. (2017). The Personality Profile of Tinnitus Sufferers and a Nontinnitus Control Group. *Journal of the American Academy of Audiology*, 28, pp. 271–282. https://doi.org/10.3766/jaaa.15103

Dyke, P. (2013). *A clear view: Identifying Australians who live with deafblindness and dual sensory loss.* Senses Australia. [Online] Available at: www.senseswa.com.au/wp-content/uploads/2016/01/a-clear-view---senses-australia.pdf

Dykstra, P. A., van Tilburg, T. G., & de Jong Gierveld, J. (2005). Changes in older adult loneliness. *Research on Aging, 27*(6), 725–747. https://doi.org/10.1177/0164027505279712

Eagar, K., Owen, A., Williams, K., Westera, A., Marosszeky, N., England, R. and Morris, D. (2007). Effective caring: A synthesis of the international evidence on carer needs and interventions. Centre for Health Service Development, University of Wollongong. [Online] Available at: https://ro.uow.edu.au/chsd/27/

Eggins, S., Slade, D. and Geddes, F. (2016). *Effective Communication in Clinical Handover: From Research to Practice.* Berlin: Walter de Gruyter GmbH & Co. KG.

Erber, N. P. and Scherer, S. C. (1999). Sensory Loss and Communication Difficulties in the Elderly. *Australasian Journal on Ageing*, 18(1), pp. 4–9. https://doi.org/10.1111/j.1741-6612.1999.tb00079.x

Fellinger, J., Holzinger, D., Dirmhirn, A., van Dijk, J. and Goldberg, D. (2009). Failure to Detect Deaf-Blindness in a Population of People with Intellectual Disability. *Journal of Intellectual Disability Research*, 53(10), pp. 874–881. https://doi.org/10.1111/j.1365-2788.2009.01205.x

Ffytche, D. H., Creese, B., Politis, M., Chaudhuri, K. R., Weintraub, D., Ballard, C. and Aarsland, D. (2017). 'The psychosis spectrum in Parkinson disease', *Nature reviews. Neurology*, 13(2), pp. 81–95.

Foreman, J., Xie, J., Keel, S., van Wijngaarden, P., Sandhu, S. S., Ang, G. S., Fan Gaskin, J., Crowston, J., Bourne, R., Taylor, H. R. and Dirani, M. (2017). The Prevalence and Causes of Vision Loss in Indigenous and Non-Indigenous Australians: The National Eye Health Survey. *Ophthalmology*, 124(12), pp. 1743–1752. https://doi.org/10.1016/j.ophtha.2017.06.001

Fraser, S. A., Beeman, I., Southall, K. and Wittich, W. (2019). Stereotyping as a Barrier to the Social Participation of Older Adults with Low Vision: A Qualitative Focus Group Study. *BMJ Open*, 9(9), Article e029940. https://doi.org/10.1136/bmjopen-2019-029940

Fricker, M. (2007). *Epistemic injustice: power and the ethics of knowing*, Oxford University Press, Oxford.

Fukuyama, F. (2020). The Pandemic and Political Order. Foreign Affairs. [Online] Available at: www.foreignaffairs.com/articles/world/2020-06-09/pandemic-and-political-order

GBD 2016 Disease and Injury Incidence and Prevalence Collaborators. (2017). Global, Regional, and National Incidence, Prevalence, and Years Lived with Disability for 328 Diseases and Injuries for 195 Countries, 1990–2016: A Systematic Analysis for the Global Burden of Disease Study 2016. *The Lancet*, 390(10100), pp. 1211–1259. https://doi.org/10.1016/s0140-6736(17)32154-2

Gheorghe, D. C. and Zamfir-Chiru-Anton, A. (2015). Complications in Cochlear Implant Surgery. *Journal of Medicine and Life*, 8(3), p. 329.

Gledhill, K. and Baird, N. (2023). Ensuring a Disability Perspective in Disaster Law: The Contribution of the Committee on the Rights of Persons with Disabilities. *Yearbook of International Disaster Law Online*, 4(1), pp. 432–464. https://doi.org/10.1163/26662531_00401_021

Gopinath, B., Schneider, J., McMahon, C. M., Burlutsky, G., Leeder, S. R. and Mitchell, P. (2013). Dual Sensory Impairment in Older Adults Increases the Risk of Mortality: A Population-Based Study. *PLoS One*, 8(3), Article e55054. https://doi.org/10.1371/journal.pone.0055054

Gordon, K. D. and Felfeli, T. (2018). Family Physician Awareness of Charles Bonnet Syndrome. *Family Practice*, 35(5), pp. 595–598.

Granovetter, M. S. (1973). The Strength of Weak Ties. *American Journal of Sociology*, 78(6), pp. 1360–1380. https://doi.org/10.1086/225469

Guthrie, D. M., & Poss, J. W. (2013). Development of a case-mix funding system for adults with combined vision and hearing loss.

BMC Health Services Research, *13*(1), Article 137. https://doi.org/10.1186/1472-6963-13-137

Guthrie, D. M., Declercq, A., Finne-Soveri, H., Fries, B. E. and Hirdes, J. P. (2016). The Health and Well-Being of Older Adults with Dual Sensory Impairment (DSI) in Four Countries. *PLoS One*, 11(5), Article e0155073. https://doi.org/10.1371/journal.pone.0155073

Guthrie, D. M., Davidson, J. G. S., Williams, N., Campos, J., Hunter, K., Mick, P., Orange, J. B., Pichora-Fuller, M. K., Phillips, N. A., Savundranayagam, M. Y. and Wittich, W. (2018). Combined Impairments in Vision, Hearing and Cognition are Associated with Greater Levels of Functional and Communication Difficulties than Cognitive Impairment Alone: Analysis of interRAI Data for Home Care and Long-Term Care Recipients in Ontario. *PloS one*, 13(2), e0192971. https://doi.org/10.1371/journal.pone.0192971

Guthrie, D.M., Williams, N. and Jaiswal, A. (2022). Prevalence of Sensory Impairments in Home Care and Long-Term Care Using interRAI Data From Across Canada. *BMC Geriatr* 22, 944. https://doi.org/10.1186/s12877-022-03671-7

Hajek, A. and König, H. H. (2020). Dual Sensory Impairment and Healthcare Use: Findings From a Nationally Representative Sample. *Geriatrics & Gerontology International*, 20(6), pp. 602–606. https://doi.org/10.1111/ggi.13929

Hawkley, L. C. and Capitanio, J. P. (2015). Perceived Social Isolation, Evolutionary Fitness and Health Outcomes: A Lifespan Approach. *Philosophical Transactions of the Royal Society B: Biological Sciences*, 370(1669), 20140114.

Hedges, T. R. (2007). Charles Bonnet, His Life, and His Syndrome. *Survey of Ophthalmology*, 52(1), pp. 111–114. https://doi.org/10.1016/j.survophthal.2006.10.007

Heine, C. and Browning, C. J. (2002). Communication and Psychosocial Consequences of Sensory Loss in Older Adults: Overview and Rehabilitation Directions. *Disability and Rehabilitation*, 24(15), pp. 763–773. https://doi.org/10.1080/09638280210129162

Heine, C. and Browning, C. J. (2004). The Communication and Psychosocial Perceptions of Older Adults With Sensory Loss: A Qualitative Study. *Ageing and Society*, 24(1), pp. 113– 130. https://doi.org/10.1017/S0144686X03001491

Heine, C. and Browning, C. (2015). Dual Sensory Loss in Older Adults: A Systematic Review. *The Gerontologist*, 55(5), pp. 913– 928. https://doi.org/10.1093/geront/gnv074

Heine, C., Gong, C. H. and Browning, C. (2019). Dual Sensory Loss, Mental Health, and Wellbeing of Older Adults Living in China. *Frontiers in Public Health*, 7, Article 92. https://doi.org/10.3389/fpubh.2019.00092

Henry, J. A., Reavis, K. M., Griest, S. E., Thielman, E. J., Theodoroff, S. M., Grush, L. D. and Carlson, K. F. (2020). Tinnitus. *Otolaryngologic Clinics of North America*, 53(4), pp. 481–499. https://doi.org/10.1016/j.otc.2020.03.002

Hersh, M. (2013). Deafblind People, Communication, Independence, and Isolation. *Journal of Deaf Studies and Deaf Education*, 18(4), pp. 446–463. https://doi.org/10.1093/deafed/ent022

Hirvonen, M., Ojala, R., Korhonen, P., Haataja, P., Eriksson, K., Gissler, M., Luukkaala, T. and Tammela, O. (2018). Visual and Hearing Impairments After Preterm Birth. *Pediatrics*, 142(2), e20173888. https://doi.org/10.1542/peds.2017-3888

Hofsöe, S. M., Lehane, C. M., Wittich, W., Hilpert, P. and Dammeyer, J. (2019). Interpersonal Communication and Psychological Well-Being Among Couples Coping With Sensory Loss: The Mediating Role of Perceived Spouse Support. *Journal of Social and Personal Relationships*, 36(8), pp. 2323–2344. https://doi.org/10.1177/0265407518787933

Hoffman, H. J. and Reed, G. W. (2004). Epidemiology of tinnitus. *Tinnitus: Theory and management*, 16-41

Holt-Lunstad, J. (2017). The Potential Public Health Relevance of Social Isolation and Loneliness: Prevalence, Epidemiology, and Risk Factors. *The Public Policy and Aging Report*, 27(4), pp. 127–130. https://doi.org/10.1093/ppar/prx030

Holt-Lunstad, J. (2018). Why social relationships are important for physical health: A systems approach to understanding and modifying risk and protection. *Annual Review of Psychology*, *69*, 437–458. https://doi.org/10.1146/annurev-psych-122216-011902

Holt-Lunstad, J. and Perissinotto, C. (2023). Social Isolation and Loneliness as Medical Issues. *New England Journal of Medicine*, 388(3), pp. 193–195.

Holt-Lunstad, J., Robles, T. F. and Sbarra, D. A. (2017). Advancing Social Connection as a Public Health Priority in the United States. *American Psychologist*, 72(6), pp. 517–530. https://doi.org/10.1037/amp0000103

Holt-Lunstad, J., Smith, T. B., Baker, M., Harris, T. and Stephenson, D. (2015). Loneliness and Social Isolation as Risk Factors for Mortality: A Meta-Analytic Review. *Perspectives on Psychological Science*, 10(2), pp. 227–237. https://doi.org/10.1177/1745691614568352

Holt-Lunstad, J., Smith, T. B. and Layton, J. B. (2010). Social Relationships and Mortality Risk: A Meta-Analytic Review. *PLoS Medicine*, 7(7), Article e1000316. https://doi.org/10.1371/journal.pmed.100031

Horowitz, A., Goodman, C. R. and Reinhardt, J. P. (2004). Congruence Between Disabled Elders and Their Primary Caregivers. *The Gerontologist*, 44(4), pp. 532–542. https://doi.org/10.1093/geront/44.4.532

House of Representatives Standing Committee on Health, Aged Care and Sport. (2017). *Still waiting to be heard...Report on the Inquiry into the Hearing Health and Wellbeing of Australia.* CANBERRA, Australian Capital Territory: Department of the Senate. https://parlinfo.aph.gov.au/parlInfo/search/display/display.w3p;query=Id%3A%22committees%2Freportrep%2F024048%2F0000%22

Hussain, S. F., Raza, Z., Cash, A. T., Zampieri, T., Mazzoli, R. A., Kardon, R. H. and Gomes, R.S. (2021). Traumatic Brain Injury and Sight Loss in Military and Veteran Populations–A Review. *Military Medical Research*, 8(1), pp. 1–14.

Huddle, M. G., Deal, J. A., Swenor, B., Genther, D. J. and Lin, F. R. (2016). Association Between Dual Sensory Impairment, Hospitalization, and Burden of Disease. *Journal of the American Geriatrics Society*, 64(8), pp. 1735–1737. https://doi.org/10.1111/jgs.14210

Inouye, S. K., Westendorp, R. G. and Saczynski, J. S. (2014). Delirium in Elderly People. *The Lancet*, 383(9920), pp. 911–922.

Jaiswal, A., Aldersey, H., Wittich, W., Mirza, M. and Finlayson, M. (2018). Participation Experiences of People with Deafblindness or Dual Sensory Loss: A Scoping Review of Global Deafblind Literature. *PLoS One*, 13(9), Article e0203772. https://doi.org/10.1371/journal.pone.0203772

Jaiswal, A., Fraser, S. and Wittich, W. (2020). Barriers and Facilitators that Influence Social Participation in Older Adults with Dual Sensory Impairment. *Frontiers in Education*, 5, Article 127. https://doi.org/10.3389/feduc.2020.00127

Jones, L., Ditzel-Finn, L., Enoch, J. and Moosajee, M. (2021). An Overview of Psychological and Social Factors in Charles Bonnet Syndrome. *Therapeutic Advances in Ophthalmology*, 13, 25158414211034715. https://doi.org/10.1177/2515841421 1034715

Kahn, R. L. and Antonucci, T. C. (1980). Convoys over the life course: Attachment, roles, and social support. In: P. B. Baltes and O. G. Brim, eds., *Life-Span Development and Behavior*. Academic Press, pp. 253–286.

Kelley, D. E., Lewis, M. A. and Southwell, B. G. (2017). Perceived Support From a Caregiver's Social Ties Predicts Subsequent Care-Recipient Health. *Preventive Medicine Reports*, 8, pp. 108–111. https://doi.org/10.1016/j.pmedr.2017.08.001

Kendig, H., Gong, C. H., Cannon, L. and Browning, C. (2017). Preferences and Predictors of Aging in Place: Longitudinal Evidence From Melbourne, Australia. *Journal of Housing for the Elderly*, 31(3), pp. 259–271. https://doi.org/10.1080/02763 893.2017.1280582

Kennard C. (2018). Charles Bonnet Syndrome – Disturbing 'Playthings of the Brain'. *Practical Neurology*, 18(6), pp. 434–435. https://doi.org/10.1136/practneurol-2018-002046

Khan, J. C., Shahid, H., Thurlby, D. A, Yates J. R. W. and Moore, A. T. (2008). Charles Bonnet syndrome in age-related macular degeneration: the nature and frequency of images in subjects with end-stage disease. *Ophthalmic Epidemiol.*, 15(3), pp. 202–8. https://doi.org/10.1080/09286580801939320

Kiely, K. M., Mortby, M. E. and Anstey, K. J. (2020). Third-Party Impact of Dual Sensory Loss on Neuropsychiatric Symptom-Related Distress Among Friends and Family. *Gerontology*, 66(4), pp. 351–361. https://doi.org/10.1159/000507856

Kong, H. H., Shin, K. and Won, C. W. (2023). Association of Dual Sensory Impairment with Declining Physical Function in Community-Dwelling Older Adults. *International Journal of Environmental Research and Public Health*, 20(4), p. 3546. https://doi.org/10.3390/ijerph20043546

Kwon, H. J., Kim, J.-S., Kim, Y.-J., Kwon, S.-J. and Yu, J.-N. (2015). Sensory Impairment and Health-Related Quality of Life. *Iranian Journal of Public Health*, 44(6), pp. 772–782.

Lahtinen, R. & Palmer, R. (1994). Communication with Usher People, Practical Ideas for the Family and Professional. DEAFBLIND EDUCATION. IAEDB publication, July, 7-9.

Lahtinen, R. (2008). *Haptices and haptemes. A case study of developmental process in social-haptic communication of acquired deafblind people*. Doctoral theses. University of Helsinki.

Lahtinen, R., Palmer, R. and Lahtinen, M. (2010). *Environmental Description for Visually and Dual Sensory Impaired People*. Helsinki: Art-Print Oy.

Lahtinen, R., Palmer, R. & Tuomaala, S. (2016). Dbl Review. Using haptices in health care settings. 56/2016, 18-19.

Lahtinen, R. and Palmer, R. (2005). *The Body Story: Creating Musical Images Through Touch (CMIT)*. Tampere, Finland: City-Offset.

Lang, E. V. (2012). A Better Patient Experience Through Better Communication. *Journal of Radiology Nursing*, 31(4), pp, 114–119. https://doi.org/10.1016/j.jradnu.2012.08.001

Larsen, F. A. and Damen, S. (2014). Definitions of Deafblindness and Congenital Deafblindness. *Research in Developmental Disabilities*, 35(10), pp. 2568–2576. https://doi.org/10.1016/j.ridd.2014.05.029

Leach and Scully 2020 Lejeune, B. J. (2010). Aging With a Dual Sensory Loss: Thoughts From Consumer Focus Groups. *AER Journal: Research and Practice in Visual Impairment and Blindness*, 3(4), pp. 146–152.

Lee E, and Brennan, M. (2006) Stress constellations and coping styles of older adults with age-related visual impairment. *Health Soc Work*. 31: 289–298

Lehane, C. M., Dammeyer, J. and Elsass, P. (2017). Sensory Loss and Its Consequences For Couples' Psychosocial and Relational Wellbeing: An Integrative Review. *Aging and Mental Health*, 21(4), pp. 337–347. https://doi.org/10.1080/13607863.2015.1132675

Lehane, C. M., Elsass, P., Hovaldt, H. B. and Dammeyer, J. (2018). A Relationship-Focused Investigation of Spousal Psychological Adjustment to Dual-Sensory Loss. *Aging & Mental Health*, 22(3), pp. 397–404. https://doi.org/10.1080/13607863.2016.1268091

Lehane, C. M., Hofsöe, S. M., Wittich, W. and Dammeyer, J. (2018). Mental Health and Spouse Support Among Older Couples Living With Sensory Loss. *Journal of Aging and Health*, 30(8), pp. 1205–1223. https://doi.org/10.1177/0898264317713135

Lejeune, B. J. (2010). Aging With a Dual Sensory Loss: Thoughts From Consumer Focus Groups. *AER Journal: Research and Practice in Visual Impairment and Blindness*, 3(4), pp. 146–152.

Levi, M. (2023) *We Need to Talk About Ageing*. Australia: Hachette.

Lin, M. Y., Gutierrez, P. R., Stone, K. L., Yaffe, K., Ensrud, K. E., Fink, H. A., Sarkisian, C. A., Coleman, A. L. and Mangione, C. M. (2004). Vision Impairment and Combined Vision and Hearing Impairment Predict Cognitive and Functional Decline in Older Women.

Journal of the American Geriatrics Society, 52(12), pp. 1996–2002. https://doi.org/10.1111/j.1532-5415.2004.52554.x

Livingston, G., Huntley, J., Sommerlad, A., Ames, D., Ballard, C., Banerjee, S., Brayne, C., Burns, A., Cohen-Mansfield, J., Cooper, C., Costafreda, S. G., Dias, A., Fox, N., Gitlin, L. N., Howard, R., Kales, H. C., Kivimäki, M., Larson, E. B., Ogunniyi, A., Orgeta, V., Ritchie, K., Rockwood, K., Sampson, E. L., Samus, Q., Schneider, L. S., Selbæk, G., Teri, L. and Mukadam, N. (2020). Dementia Prevention, Intervention, and Care: 2020 Report of the Lancet Commission. *Lancet*, 396(10248), pp. 413–446. https://doi.org/10.1016/S0140-6736(20)30367-6

Lopes, A. and Sales, P. (2016). A Case Report of Charles Bonnet Syndrome – The Silent Doubt: Am I Crazy? *European Psychiatry*, 33, P. S471. 10.1016/j.eurpsy.2016.01.1717.

Luo, Y., Hawkley, L. C., Waite, L. J., & Cacioppo, J. T. (2012). Loneliness, health, and mortality in old age: A national longitudinal study. *Social Science & Medicine, 74*(6), 907–914. https://doi.org/10.1016/j.socscimed.2011.11.028

Mah, H. Y., Ishak, W. S. and Abd Rahman, M. H. (2020). Prevalence and Risk Factors of Dual Sensory Impairment Among Community-Dwelling Older Adults in Selangor: A Secondary Data Analysis. *Geriatrics & Gerontology International*, 20(10), pp. 911–916. https://doi.org/10.1111/ggi.14011

Maharani, A., Dawes, P., Nazroo, J., Tampubolon, G., & Pendleton, N. (2020). Associations between self-reported sensory impairment and risk of cognitive decline and impairment in the Health and Retirement Study cohort. *The Journals of Gerontology. Series B, Psychological Sciences and Social Sciences*, 75(6), 1230–1242. https://doi.org/10.1093/geronb/gbz043

Mancini, P. C.., Tyler, R.. S., Smith, S., Ji, H., Perreau, A. and Mohr, A. M. (2019). Tinnitus: How partners can help?. *American journal of audiology*, 28(1), pp. 85-94. https://doi.org/0.1044/2018_AJA-18-0046

Maresova, P., Javanmardi, E., Barakovic, S. Barakovic Husic, J., Tomsone, S., Krejcar, O. and Kuca, K. (2019) Consequences of

Chronic Diseases and Other Limitations Associated With Old Age – A Scoping Review. *BMC Public Health*, 19, Article 1431 https://doi.org/10.1186/s12889-019-7762-5

Marmamula, S., Kumbham, T. R., Modepalli, S. B., Barrenkala, N. R., Yellapragada, R. and Shidhaye, R. (2021). Depression, Combined Visual and Hearing Impairment (Dual Sensory Impairment): A Hidden Multi-Morbidity Among the Elderly in Residential Care in India. *Scientific Reports*, 11(1), Article 16189. https://doi.org/10.1038/s41598-021-95576-5

Maxmen, A. (2019). The Devastating Biological Effects of Homelessness. *Nature*. [Online] Available at: www.nature.com/articles/d41586-019-01573-0

McCormack, A., Edmondson-Jones, M., Somerset, S., et. al. (2016). A Systematic Review of the Reporting of Tinnitus Prevalence and Severity. Hear Res, 337, pp. 70–79.

McFerran, D. J., Stockdale, D., Holme, R., et. al. (2019). Why is There No Cure For Tinnitus? *Front Neurosci*, 13, p. 802.

Menon, G. J. (2005). Complex Visual Hallucinations in The Visually Impaired: A Structured History-Taking Approach. *Archives of Ophthalmology (Chicago, Ill.: 1960)*, 123(3), pp. 349–355. https://doi.org/10.1001/archopht.123.3.349

Menon, G. J., Rahman, I., Menon, S. J. and Dutton, G.N. (2003). Complex visual hallucinations in the visually impaired: the Charles Bonnet Syndrome. *Survey of ophthalmology*, 48(1), pp.58-72.

Miller K, Shoemaker M, Willyard J, Addison P. (2008) Providing care for elderly parents: A structural approach to family caregiver identity. *Journal of Family Communication* 2008; 8: 19–43.

Mick, P., Parfyonov, M., Wittich, W., Phillips, N., Guthrie, D. and Pichora-Fuller, M. K. (2018). Associations Between Sensory Loss and Social Networks, Participation, Support, and Loneliness: Analysis of the Canadian Longitudinal Study on Aging. *Canadian Family Physician*, 64(1), pp. e33–e41.

Mick, P. T., Hämäläinen, A., Kolisang, L., Pichora-Fuller, M. K., Phillips, N., Guthrie, D. and Wittich, W. (2021). The Prevalence of Hearing, Vision, and Dual Sensory Loss in Older Canadians: An Analysis of Data From the Canadian Longitudinal Study on Aging. *Canadian Journal on Aging*, 40(1), pp. 1–22. https://doi.org/10.1017/S0714980820000070

Minakaran, N., Soorma, T., Bronstein, A. M., & Plant, G. T. (2019). Charles Bonnet syndrome and periodic alternating nystagmus: moving visual hallucinations. *Neurology*, *92*(10), e1072-e1075.

Moller, A. C. and Deci, E. L. (2005). The concept of competence: A starting place for understanding intrinsic motivation and self-determined extrinsic motivation. In: A. J. Elliot and C. S. Dweck, eds., *Handbook of Competence and Motivation*. Guilford Publications, pp. 579–597.

Monin, J. K., Levy, B., Doyle, M., Schulz, R. and Kershaw, T. (2019). The Impact of Both Spousal Caregivers' and Care Recipients' Health on Relationship Satisfaction in the Caregiver Health Effects Study. *Journal of Health Psychology*, 24(12), pp. 1744–1755. https://doi.org/10.1177/1359105317699682

Moring, J. C., Peterson, A. L. and Kanzler, K. E. (2018). Tinnitus, Traumatic Brain Injury, and Posttraumatic Stress Disorder in the Military. *International Journal of Behavioral Medicine*, 25, pp. 312–321.

Nair, A. G., Nair, A. G., Shah, B. R. and Gandhi, R. A. (2015). Charles Bonnet Syndrome Revisited. *Psychogeriatrics*, 15, pp. 204–208. https://doi.org/10.1111/psyg.12091

Newall, P., Mitchell, P., Sindhusake, D., Golding, Wigney, Hartley, Smith, & Birtles. (2001). Tinnitus in Older People: It is a Widespread Problem. *The Hearing Journal*, 54, pp. 14–18.

Nieman, E. (2018). Charles Bonnet Syndrome. *Pract Neurol*. 18(6), pp. 518–519. https://doi.org/10.1136/practneurol-2018-002023

Niazi, S., Krogh Nielsen, M., Singh, A., Sørensen, T. L. and Subhi, Y. (2020). Prevalence of Charles Bonnet Syndrome in Patients

With Age-Related Macular Degeneration: Systematic Review and Meta-Analysis. *Acta Ophthalmologica*, 98(2), pp. 121–131. https://doi.org/10.1111/aos.14287

Nikolaraizi, M., Argyropoulos, V., Papazafiri, M. and Kofidou, C. (2021). Promoting Accessible and Inclusive Education on Disaster Risk Reduction: The Case of Students With Sensory Disabilities. *International Journal of Inclusive Education.* https://doi.org/10.1080/13603116.2020.1862408

Palmer, R. & Lahtinen, R. (1994). Communication with Usher People. Deafblind Education, July-December, 1994, p7–9.

Palmer, R. and Lahtinen, R. (2013). History of Social-Haptic Communication. *Deafblind International Review*, pp. 68–71.

Pang, L. (2016). Hallucinations Experienced by Visually Impaired: Charles Bonnet Syndrome. *Optometry and Vision Science: Official Publication of the American Academy of Optometry*, 93(12), pp. 1466–1478. https://doi.org/10.1097/OPX.0000000000000959

Pani-Harreman, K. E., Bours, G. J. J. W., Zander, I., Kempen, G. I. J. M. and van Duren, J. M. A. (2021). Definitions, Key Themes and Aspects of "Ageing in Place": A Scoping Review. *Ageing & Society*, 41(9), pp. 2026–2059. https://doi.org/10.1017/S0144686X20000094

Paradies, Y. (2018). Whither standpoint theory in a post-truth world? *Cosmopolitan Civil Societies, an Interdisciplinary Journal*, 10(2), pp. 119-29 https://doi.org/10.5130/ccs.v10i2.5980

Pavey, S., Douglas, G., Hodges, L., Bodsworth, S. and Clare, I. (2009). *The needs of older people with acquired hearing and sight loss* (Research findings). Thomas Pocklington Trust.

Pérez-Garín, D., Recio, P., & Molero, F. (2021). Consequences of perceived personal and group discrimination against people with hearing and visual impairments. *International Journal of Environmental Research and Public Health*, 18(17), Article 9064. https://doi.org/10.3390/ijerph18179064

Pirkis, J., Pfaff, J., Williamson, M., Tyson, O., Stocks, N., Goldney, R., Draper, B., Snowdon, J., Lautenschlager, N. and Almeida, O. P. (2009). The Community Prevalence of Depression in Older Australians. *J Affect Disord*, 115(1–2), pp. 54–61. https://doi.org/10.1016/j.jad.2008.08.014

Potts, A., Bednarek, M. A., & Watharow, A. (2023). Super, social, medical: Person-first and identity-first representations of disabled people in Australian newspapers, 2000–2019. *Discourse & Society*, 09579265231156504.

Randall, A. K. and Bodenmann, G. (2009). The Role of Stress on Close Relationships and Marital Satisfaction. *Clinical Psychology Review*, 29(2), pp. 105–115. https://doi.org/10.1016/j.cpr.2008.10.004

Reed, N. S., Assi, L., Pedersen, E., Alshabasy, Y., Deemer, A., Deal, J. A., Willink, A. and Swenor, B. K. (2020). Accompaniment to Healthcare Visits: The Impact of Sensory Impairment. *BMC Health Services Research*, 20(1), Article 990. https://doi.org/10.1186/s12913-020-05829-8

Rohan, K. J., Roecklein, K. A., Tierney Lindsey, K., Johnson, L. G., Lippy, R. D., Lacy, T. J. and Barton, F. B. (2007). A Randomized Controlled Trial of Cognitive-Behavioral Therapy, Light Therapy, and Their Combination For Seasonal Affective Disorder. *J Consult Clin Psychol*, 75(3), pp. 489–500. https://doi.org/10.1037/0022-006X.75.3.489

Rosengren, K., Buttigieg, S. C., Badanta, B., & Carlstrom, E. (2023). Diffusion of person-centred care within 27 European countries–interviews with managers, officials, and researchers at the micro, meso, and macro levels. *Journal of Health Organization and Management*, *37*(1), 17-34.

Russell, D., McLaughlin, J. and Demko, R. (2018). Barrier-Free Emergency Communication Access and Alerting System Research Report. *Canadian Hearing Society*. [Online] Available at: www.chs.ca/sites/default/files/barrier-free_emergency_communication_access_and_alerting_system_research_report.pdf

Salazar, J. W., Meisel, K.., Smith, E. R., Quiggle, A., McCoy, D. B., Amans M. R.. (2019). 'Depression in Patients with Tinnitus: A Systematic Review', *Otolaryngology–head and neck surgery: official journal of American Academy of Otolaryngology-Head and Neck Surgery.* 161(1), pp. 28-35. doi: https://doi.org/10.1177/0194599819835178

Scarinci, N., Worrall, L. and Hickson, L. (2008). The Effect of Hearing Impairment in Older People on the Spouse. *International Journal of Audiology*, 47(3), pp. 141–151. https://doi.org/10.1080/149920 20701689696

Scarinci, N., Worrall, L. and Hickson, L. (2009). The ICF and Third-Party Disability: Its Application to Spouses of Older People With Hearing Impairment. *Disabil. Rehabil.* 31, pp. 2088–2100

Schneider, J. M., Gopinath, B., McMahon, C. M., Leeder, S. R., Mitchell, P. and Wang, J. J. (2011). Dual Sensory Impairment in Older Age. *Journal of Aging and Health*, 23(8), pp. 1309–1324. https://doi.org/10.1177/0898264311408418

Schneider, J., Gopinath, B., McMahon, C., Teber, E., Leeder, S. R., Wang, J. J. and Mitchell, P. (2012). Prevalence and 5-Year Incidence of Dual Sensory Impairment in an Older Australian Population. *Annals of Epidemiology*, 22(4), pp. 295–301. https://doi.org/ 10.1016/j.annepidem.2012.02.004

Shakarchi, A. F., Assi, L., Ehrlich, J. R., Deal, J. A., Reed, N. S. and Swenor, B. K. (2020). Dual Sensory Impairment and Perceived Everyday Discrimination in the United States. *JAMA Ophthalmology*, 138(12), pp. 1227–1233. https://doi.org/10.1001/jamaophthal mol.2020.3982

Shakespeare, T. (2021). Triple Jeopardy: Disabled People and the COVID-19 Pandemic. *The Lancet*, 397(10282), pp. 1331–1333.

Sharif, A., McCall, A. L. and Bolante, K. R. (2022). Should I Say "Disabled People" or "People with Disabilities"? Language Preferences of Disabled People Between Identity- and Person-First Language. *In Proceedings of the 24th International ACM SIGACCESS Conference on Computers and Accessibility (ASSETS '22).*

Association for Computing Machinery, New York, NY, USA, Article 10, 1–18. https://doi.org/10.1145/3517428.3544813

Sherman-Morris, K., Pechacek, T., Griffin, D. and Senkbeil, J. (2020). Tornado Warning Awareness, Information Needs and the Barriers to Protective Action of Individuals Who are Blind. *International Journal of Disaster Risk Reduction*, 50. https://doi.org/10.1016/j.ijdrr.2020.101709

Shu, C.-C., Hsu, B., Cumming, R. G., Blyth, F. M., Waite, L. M., Le Couteur, D. G., Handelsman, D. J. and Naganathan, V. (2019). Caregiving and All-Cause Mortality in Older Men 2005–15: The Concord Health and Ageing in Men Project. *Age and Ageing*, 48(4), pp. 571–576. https://doi.org/10.1093/ageing/afz039

Sindhusake, D., Golding, M., Newall, P., Rubin, G., Jakobsen, K., Mitchell, P. (2003). Risk Factors for Tinnitus in a Population of Older Adults: The Blue Mountains Hearing Study. *Ear and Hearing* 24(6), 501-507. https://doi.org/10.1097/01.AUD.0000100204.08771.3D

Simcock, P. (2017). Ageing With a Unique Impairment: A Systematically Conducted Review of Older Deafblind People's Experiences. *Ageing & Society*, 37(8), pp. 1703–1742. https://doi.org/10.1017/S0144686X16000520

Simcock, P. and Castle, R. (2016). *Social Work and Disability*. John Wiley & Sons.

Simcock, P., Manthorpe, J. and Tinker, A. (2023). A Salutogenesis Approach to Ageing with Impairment: The Managing and Coping Experiences of Older People Ageing with Deafblindness. *Ageing & Society*, 43(12), pp. 2957–2982.

Simcock, P. and Wittich, W. (2019). Are Older Deafblind People Being Left Behind? A Narrative Review of Literature on Deafblindness Through the Lens of the United Nations Principles for Older People. *Journal of Social Welfare & Family Law*, 41(3), pp. 339–357. https://doi.org/10.1080/09649069.2019.1627088

Simning, A., Fox, M. L., Barnett, S. L., Sorensen, S. and Conwell, Y. (2019). Depressive and Anxiety Symptoms in Older Adults with Auditory, Vision, and Dual Sensory Impairment. *J Aging Health*, 31(8), pp. 1353–1375. https://doi.org/10.1177/089826431 8781123

Singh, A., Subhi, Y. and Sørensen, T. L. (2014). Low Awareness of the Charles Bonnet Syndrome in Patients Attending a Retinal Clinic. *Dan Med J*, 61(2), A4770.

Slade, D., Manidis, M., McGregor, J., Sheeres, H., Chandler, E., SteinParbury, J., Dunston, R., Herke, M. and Matthiessen, C. M. I. M. (2015). *Communicating in Hospital Emergency Departments*. Heidelberg, Germany: Springer.

Smith, S. L., Bennett, L. W. and Wilson, R. H. (2008). Prevalence and Characteristics of Dual Sensory Impairment (hearing and vision) in a Veteran Population. *Journal of Rehabilitation Research & Development*, 45(4), pp. 597–609. https://doi.org/10.1682/ jrrd.2007.02.0023

Southall, K., Gagné, J.-P. and Jennings, M. B. (2010). Stigma: A Negative and a Positive Influence on Help-Seeking for Adults With Acquired Hearing Loss. *International Journal of Audiology*, 49(11), pp. 804–814. https://doi.org/10.3109/14992027.2010.498447

Strawbridge, W. J., Wallhagen, M. I., Shema, S. J. and Kaplan, G. A. (2000). Negative Consequences of Hearing Impairment in Old Age: A Longitudinal Analysis. *The Gerontologist*, 40(3), pp. 320–326. https://doi.org/10.1093/geront/40.3.320

Stephens, C., Alpass, F., Towers, A. and Stevenson, B. (2011). The Effects of Types of Social Networks, Perceived Social Support, and Loneliness on the Health of Older People: Accounting for the Social Context. *Journal of Aging and Health*, 23(6), pp. 887–911. https://doi.org/10.1177/0898264311400189

Sutherland, K., Hindmarsh, D., Moran, K. and Levesque, J. (2017). Disparities in Experiences and Outcomes of Hospital Care Between Aboriginal and Non-Aboriginal Patients in New South Wales. *Medical Journal of Australia*, 207(1), pp. 17–18. https://doi. org/10.5694/mja16.00777

Swenor, B. K., Ramulu, P. Y., Willis, J. R., Friedman, D., & Lin, F. R. (2013). The prevalence of concurrent hearing and vision impairment in the United States. *JAMA Internal Medicine*, *173*(4), 312–313. https://doi.org/10.1001/jamainternmed.2013.1880

Takahashi, N. (2019). Accessibility For People With Deafblindness When Getting Medical Services. In: *Deafblind International World Conference*, 12–16 August, Gold Coast, Australia.

Takayama, K., Craig, L., Cooper, A. and Stokar, H. (2022). Exploring Deaf Students' Disaster Awareness and Preparedness in U.S. Higher Education Settings: Implications For University-Level DRR Policy and Programming. *International Journal of Disaster Risk Reduction*, 83. https://doi.org/10.1016/j.ijdrr.2022.103409

Theodoroff, S. M., Lewis, M. S., Folmer, R. L., Henry, J. A. and Carlson, K. F. (2015). Hearing Impairment and Tinnitus: Prevalence, Risk Factors, and Outcomes in US Service Members and Veterans Deployed to the Iraq and Afghanistan Wars. *Epidemiologic Reviews*, 37(1), pp. 71–85.

Tian, L., Bashir, N. Y., Chasteen, A. L. and Rule, N. O. (2020). The Effect of Age-Stigma Concealment on Social Evaluations. *Basic and Applied Social Psychology*, 42(4), pp. 219–234. https://doi.org/10.1080/01973533.2020.1741359

Tiwana, R., Benbow, S. M. and Kingston, P. (2016). Late Life Acquired Dual-Sensory Impairment: A Systematic Review of its Impact on Everyday Competence. *British Journal of Visual Impairment*, 34(3), pp. 203–213. https://doi.org/10.1177/0264619616648727

Trotter, C. and Baidawi, S. (2015). Older Prisoners: Challenges For Inmates and Prison Management. *Australian & New Zealand Journal of Criminology*, 48(2), pp. 200–218.

Thompson, L., & Walker, A. J. (1982). The dyad as the unit of analysis: Conceptual and methodological issues. *Journal of Marriage and the Family*, 889–900.

Tseng, Y.-C., Liu, S. H.-Y., Lou, M.-F. and Huang, G.-S. (2018). Quality of Life in Older Adults With Sensory Impairments: A Systematic

Review. *Quality of Life Research*, 27(8), pp. 1957–1971. https://doi.org/10.1007/s11136-018-1799-2

Uchino, 2006 Uchino, B. N. (2006). Social support and health: A review of physiological processes potentially underlying links to disease outcomes. *Journal of Behavioral Medicine*, *29*(4), 377–387. https://doi.org/10.1007/s10865-006-9056-5

Varma, R., Vajaranant, T. S., Burkemper, B., Wu, S., Torres, M., Hsu, C., Choudhury, F. and McKean-Cowdin, R. (2016). Visual Impairment and Blindness in Adults in the United States: Demographic and Geographic Variations From 2015 to 2050. *JAMA Ophthalmol*, 134(7), pp. 802–809. https://doi.org/10.1001/jamaophthalmol.2016.1284

Viljanen, A., Törmäkangas, T., Vestergaard, S. and Andersen-Ranberg, K. (2013). Dual Sensory Loss and Social Participation in Older Europeans. *European Journal of Ageing*, 11(2), pp. 155–167. https://doi.org/10.1007/s10433-013-0291-7

Villeneuve, M. (2021). Building a roadmap for inclusive disaster risk reduction in Australian communities. *Progress in Disaster Science*, *10*, 100166.

Villeneuve, M., Crawford, T., Yen, I., Hinitt, J., Millington, M., Dignam, M. and Gardiner, E. (2021). Disability Inclusive Disaster Risk Reduction With Culturally and Linguistically Diverse (CALD) Communities in the Hawkesbury-Nepean Region: A Co-Production Approach. *International Journal of Disaster Risk Reduction*, 63(4). https:doi.org/10.1016/j.ijdrr.2021.102430

Vukicevic, M. and Fitzmaurice, K. (2010). Butterflies and Black Lacy Patterns: The Prevalence and Characteristics of Charles Bonnet Hallucinations in an Australian Population. *Clinical & Experimental Ophthalmology*, 36(7), pp. 659–65. https://doi.org/10.1111/j.1442-9071.2008.01814.x.

Wallhagen, M. I. (1993). Perceived Control and Adaptation in Elder Caregivers: Development of an Explanatory Model. *The International Journal of Aging and Human Development*, 36(3), pp. 219–237. https://doi.org/10.2190/ba90-aqx3-t6ce-abek

Wallhagen, M. I. (2009). The Stigma of Hearing Loss. *The Gerontologist*, 50(1), pp. 66–75. https://doi.org/10.1093/geront/gnp107

Wallhagen, M. (2018). Stigma: What Does the Literature Say? *The Hearing Journal*, 71(9), pp. 14–16. https://doi.org/10.1097/01.HJ.0000546262.69563.c5

Wallhagen, M. I., Strawbridge, W. J. and Shema, S. J. (2008). The Relationship Between Hearing Impairment and Cognitive Function: A 5-Year Longitudinal Study. *Research in Gerontological Nursing*, 1(2), pp. 80–86. https://doi.org/10.3928/19404921-20080401-08

Wang, S., Quan, L., Chavarro, J. E., Slopen, N., Kubzansky, L. D., Koenen, K. C., Kang, J. H., Weisskopf, M. G., Branch-Elliman, W. and Roberts, A. L. (2022). Associations of Depression, Anxiety, Worry, Perceived Stress, and Loneliness Prior to Infection with Risk of Post-COVID-19 Conditions. *JAMA Psychiatry*, 79(11), pp. 1081–1091. https://doi.org/10.1001/jamapsychiatry.2022.2640

Watharow, A. (2019). The air that I breathe: Surviving the loss of the communication senses through narrative writing, *Life Writing*, *18*(2), 171–180. https://doi.org/10.1080/14484528.2019.1570582

Watharow, A. T. (2021). *'Not knowing what is going on': The experiences of people with deafblindness–dual sensory impairment in Australian hospitals—a mixed methods study.* Doctoral dissertation. University of Technology, Sydney, NSW.

Watharow, A. (2023). *Improving the Experience of Health Care for People Living with Sensory Disability: Knowing What is Going on.* Lived Places Publishing.

Watharow, A. and Wayland, S. (2022). Making Qualitative Research Inclusive: Methodological Insights in Disability Research. *International Journal of Qualitative Methods*, 21, 16094069221095316.

Wittich, W., Southall, K., Sikora, L., Watanabe, D. H. and Gagné, J.-P. (2013). What's in a Name: Dual Sensory Impairment or

Deafblindness? *British Journal of Visual Impairment*, 31(3), pp. 198–207. https://doi.org/10.1177/0264619613490519

World Federation of the Deafblind. (2018, September). *At risk of exclusion from CRPD and SDGs implementation: Inequality and persons with deafblindness. Initial global report on situation and rights of persons with deafblindness.* [Online] Available at: www.internationaldisabilityalliance.org/sites/default/files/wfdb_complete_initial_global_report_september_2018.pdf

World Federation of the Deafblind. (2023)

World Health Organization. (2015). *World report on ageing and health.* [Online] Available at: https://apps.who.int/iris/handle/10665/186463

World Health Organization. (2019b). *World report on vision.* [Online] Available at: www.who.int/docs/default-source/documents/publications/world-vision-report-accessible.pdf

World Health Organization. (2020). *Decade of healthy ageing: Baseline report.* [Online] Available at: https://apps.who.int/iris/bitstream/handle/10665/338677/9789240017900-eng.pdf

World Health Organization. (2021a, October 4). *Ageing and health.* [Online] Available at: www.who.int/news-room/fact-sheets/detail/ageing-and-health

World Health Organization. (2021b). *Social isolation and loneliness in older people: Advocacy brief.* [Online] Available at: www.who.int/publications/i/item/9789240030749

World Health Organization. (2021c). *World report on hearing.* [Online] Available at: www.who.int/teams/noncommunicable-diseases/sensory-functions-disability-and-rehabilitation/highlighting-priorities-for-ear-and-hearing-care

Yorgason, J. B., Almeida, D., Neupert, S. D., Spiro, A., III. and Hoffman, L. (2006). A Dyadic Examination of Daily Health Symptoms and Emotional Well-Being in Late-Life Couples. *Family Relations*, 55(5), pp. 613–624. https://doi.org/10.1111/j.1741-3729.2006.00430.x

Zarenoe, R. and Ledin, T. (2014). Quality of life in patients with tinnitus and sensorineural hearing loss. *B-ent, 10*(1), 41–51.

Zhang, Y., Ge, M., Zhao, W., Liu, Y., Xia, X., Hou, L. and Dong, B. (2020). Sensory Impairment and All-Cause Mortality Among the Oldest-Old: Findings from the Chinese Longitudinal Healthy Longevity Survey (CLHLS). *The Journal of Nutrition, Health & Aging*, 24(2), pp. 132–137. https://doi.org/10.1007/s12603-020-1319-2

Recommended further reading

The latest report on the situation of older persons with deafblindness by the WFDB (December 2023). Link here: https://wfdb.eu/wfdb-global-report-on-older-people-with-deafblindness/

Kingston, P., Benbow, S., Tiwana, R. & McGee, A. (2015) The late life acquired dual sensory impairment project. Research Findings. London: Sense.

Sense (nd) Fill in the Gaps. A checklist for assessing older deafblind people. London: Sense (I've attached this to this email).

Roberts, D., Scharf, T., Bernard, M. and Crome, P. (2007) Identification of deafblind / dual sensory impairment in older people. London: Social Care Institute for Excellence. Available here.

Sense (2015) Enjoy Life. How to Help older people with sight and hearing problems. London: Sense.

Watharow, A. (2023). *Improving the Experience of Health Care for People Living with Sensory Disability: Knowing What is Going On*. New York: Lived Places Publishing.

Russ Palmer and Riitta Lahtinen website: www.russpalmer.com/

Able Australia website: https://ableaustralia.org.au/

Riitta Lahtinen book: Environmental Description: www.opensta rts.units.it/entities/publication/19ed3e2d-cf92-4244-af41-2fc2c13b0581/details

103 Haptic Signals

Danish Society of the Deafblind, June 2010

E. Calgaro, N. Craig, L. Craig, D. Dominey-Howes, J. Allen, Silent no more: Identifying and breaking through the barriers that d/Deaf people face in responding to hazards and disasters, *International Journal of Disaster Risk Reduction*, https://doi.org/10.1016/j.ijdrr.2021.102156

Gledhill, K., & Baird, N. (2023). Ensuring a disability perspective in disaster law: The contribution of the Committee on the Rights of Persons with Disabilities. *Yearbook of International Disaster Law Online*, 4(1), 432–464. https://doi.org/10.1163/26662531_00401_021

Magda Nikolaraizi, Vassilios Argyropoulos, Maria Papazafiri & Christina Kofidou (2021). Promoting accessible and inclusive education on disaster risk reduction: The case of students with sensory disabilities. *International Journal of Inclusive Education*, https://doi.org/10.1080/13603116.2020.1862408

Debra Russell, Joe McLaughlin, Robin Demko. 2018. Barrier-free emergency communication access and alerting system research report**.**

Kathleen Sherman-Morris, Taylor Pechacek, Darrin J. Griffin, Jason Senkbeil (2020). Tornado warning awareness, information needs and the barriers to protective action of individuals who are blind. *International Journal of Disaster Risk Reduction*, Volume 50. https://doi.org/10.1016/j.ijdrr.2020.101709

Kota Takayama, Leyla Craig, Audrey Cooper, Hayley Stokar. 2022. Exploring deaf students' disaster awareness and preparedness in U.S. higher education settings: Implications for university-level DRR policy and programming.

International Journal of Disaster Risk Reduction, Volume 83. https://doi.org/10.1016/j.ijdrr.2022.103409

Michelle Villeneuve et al. (2021). Disability inclusive disaster risk reduction with culturally and linguistically diverse (CALD) communities in the Hawkesbury-Nepean region: A co-production approach. *International Journal of Disaster Risk Reduction*, 63(4). https://doi.org/10.1016/j.ijdrr.2021.102430

Index

accessibility technologies. 129, 130, 139

accidents. 46, 56

acquired DSI. 23–24, 30, 152

active transition to caring role. 100, 101

activities of daily living. 39, 47, 91, 92, 121, 122, 143

afternoon difficulties. 7

aged care facilities. 28, 33, 49, 56, 96, 120, 188

Aged Care packages. 122

ageing populations. xvii, 25, 31–32, 88, 109

ageing with DSI. 2, 19, 24, 47, 90, 188

ageing–disability intersection. 108–09

agency. 117

anxiety. 50, 73, 81, 142–43, 171

artworks, enjoying. 9

assistive devices. xvii, 41–43, 223, see also hearing aids

Auslan (Australian sign language). 188, 230

bank visits. 9

BDBD (bad deafblind day). 235–36

body language. 162

body name. 161, 166

caring; art of. 97–101; in Australia. 87–88; burden of. 119; capacity, integration of. 122–24; changing roles. 94–97; in DSI context. 89–92; dyad. 91, 95, 97, 103; empathic understanding. 98, 104; family carers. see family carers; informal versus formal. 88–89; interactions in primary care. 94; multi-layered caring roles. 96–97; safe environment. 104–05; social caring capacity. 105; social engagement. 99; social facilitation and protection. 99, 103; social isolation and effort. 92–94; social networks. 104; the way forward. 102–05

cataracts. 30, 47, 56, 64, 67

causation of DSI. 30

Charles Bonnet syndrome. 52, 63–67, 70, 145–46; causal mechanisms of. 70–71; clinical challenges. 72–75; hallucinations' nature and form. 67–70; management of. 75–78; prevalence of. 71–72; and vision loss. 67

cochlear implants. 42, 47

cognitive decline. 41, 51, 99, 116, 143–44

cognitive health. 51–52

Commonwealth Home Support Programme. 122

communication difficulties. 2, 19, 38–39; and assistive devices. 41–43; and Covid-19 pandemic. 43; and health. 39–41; and health care. 45; lack of partners. 5; and social isolation. 43–44

communication strategies. 111, 117, 128–29, 182–83; and anxiety. 142–43; basic. 132; basic supports. 132–33; breakdown. 142; and Charles Bonnet syndrome. 145–46; and cognitive decline. 143–44; and delirium. 144–45; and depression. 142–43; disruption. 11; documentation of. 181–82, 204–06, 226; during health care interactions. 118; effective. 138–41; of environmental information. 132–33; and falls. 145; for health and social care professionals. 137; and health literacy. 146–48; and hearing loss. 133–35; introducing yourself to a DSI person. 132; and low

vision. 135–36; and mortality risk. 143–44; resources. 149–50; simple strategies. 131; skills and knowledge acquisition for. 141; specific conditions, management of. 141–42; super teams. 137–38; support. 99; training modules. 149; and visual hallucinations. 145–46

congenital blindness and acquired hearing loss. 23

congenital deafness and acquired vision loss. 23

congenital deafness and blindness. 22–23

consents. 40

Covid-19 pandemic. 25, 43, 49, 70, 213

data invisibility. 48

deafblind manual alphabets. 190–203

deafferentation. 70

delirium. 52, 144–45

delusions. 60–63

depression. 50, 81, 142–43

descriptor, of DSI. 18, 19

disaster management, poor inclusion in. 49–50

disaster preparedness. 213–18

distinct disability, DSI as. 20

distress. 171

economic burden, reduction of. 41

emergency preparedness. 213–18

emergency sign. 226–27

emotions, social-haptic communication. 162

empathy. 98, 104

environment; description, social-haptic communication. 160–62; safe. 99, 104–05; threats from. 46

evening difficulties. 10–12

exclusion. 48, 50

falls. 46, 56, 145

families and carers. 57, 81–82

family carers. 33, 39, 88, 91, 94, 103, 105, 114, 118, 121, *see also* caring; active and passive transitions to caring role. 100, 101; changing roles. 94–97; developing personalised strategies. 120; empathy. 98; reliance on external networks. 123; self-care. 97, 100–01, 102; and social engagement. 91, 98, 99; and social isolation. 92, 93; and social networks. 102, 115, 119, 121; and social protection. 99

fingerspelling. 188–90, 227

First Nations peoples. 34

food safety. 46

formal care. 123

functional decline. 47

General Practitioners (GP), role of. 116–17

glaucoma. 30, 67

going to the doctor, difficulties in. 5–6

going-to-hospital kit. 208–13

guiding, social-haptic communication. 169

hallucinations. *see* Charles Bonnet Syndrome; visual hallucinations

hand-over-hand Australian sign language. 189

health and hospital encounters, preparation for. 207–13

health and social support networks, integration of. 116–19

health care access. 44; experiences of. 44; service providers. 44–45

health literacy. 146–48

hearing aids. 41–43, 51, 129

hearing loss. 133–35, *see also* tinnitus; causation of. 26–27; communication supports. 134–35; prevalence of. 25–26

homeless people. 35

hospitalisations. 13, 56, 207–13

idiosyncratic series of touch messages. 204

inclusion. 118

inclusive disaster management. 49–50

informal caring. 88

informed decision making. 53

integration of care (case study). 219–22; audiologist, visits with. 224; BDBD (bad deafblind day). 235–36; case discussion. 222–24; church ladies. 227–28; cups of tea. 225; documentation of communication strategies. 226; emergency sign. 226–27; fingerspelling. 227 health haptics. 228–29; name signs. 233–34; physical health. 232; practical supports. 224–25; resources. 234–35; risk factors. 228; short cuts messaging. 230; social connections, rebuilding. 227; social haptics. 230; social wins. 234; transitions. 225–26; travel. 231–32

interpersonal relationships. 114–16

little things, impact of. 8

loneliness. 70, 72, 107, 110, 111–12

low vision. 135; communication supports. 135–36; and food and medication safety. 46; and hallucinations. see Charles Bonnet syndrome; rehabilitation of older adults with. 109

macular degeneration. 30, 67

manual alphabets. 161, 188

medication; forcible. 11; safety. 46

mental health issues. 115

mixing in crowds, difficulty in. 3

morning difficulties. 2–7

mortality risk. 143–44

multiple disability. 33, 35, 47

mutual learning. 221

name signs. 161, 166, 185–87, 233–34

neglect. 4

neuromatrix theory. 71

Nordic definition of DSI. 21

nursing homes. 3

ontological security. 53–54; families and carers. 57; residential aged care. 56–57; unpredictable people. 54; unpredictable places. 56; unpredictable privacy. 55–56; unpredictable things. 56; unpredictable trust. 55

overnight difficulties. 12–13

passive transition to caring role. 100, 101

patient self-advocacy. 149

P-CEP (person-centred emergency planning). 214–18

personal messaging sheets. 205–06

personalised caring strategies. 120

person-centred care. 121

physical health threats; from conditions causing DSI. 47; from the environment. 46; food and medication safety. 46; from functional decline. 47

presbycusis. 30, 223

prevalence of DSI. 28–29

print on palm. 187–88, 204

prisoners. 34

privacy. 55–56, 118

professionalism, lack of. 8–9, 45

prosopometamorphopsia. 69

psychological wellbeing. 50–51, 115; cognitive health. 51–52; delirium. 52; tinnitus. 52; visual hallucinations. 52

public health threats. 48; exclusion. 50; poor inclusion in disaster management. 49–50

reciprocity. 10, 98

residential aged care. 3, 11, 56–57

safe touch zones, social-haptic communication. 155

self-stigma. 109–10

service providers. 44–45

severity of DSI. 30–31

single sensory impairment data. 24

social activities. 3, 11–12

social caring roles. 105

social engagement. 99, 110, 111

social events. 7

social facilitation and protection. 99, 103

social impact. 112–14

social isolation. 43–44, 54, 70, 92–94, 109, 111–12, 113

social networks. 102, 104; building. 122–24; capacity. 120–22; and health, integration of. 116–19; importance in older age. 110; and interpersonal relationships. 114–16; navigating health care system. 119–20

social-haptic communication. 152, 182–83, 210–11; ability of. 152–53, 154; definition of. 152; emotions. 162; entering/leaving a space. 167; environmental description. 160–62; guiding. 169; in health care. 171; history of. 153–54; name sign (body name). 166; safe touch zones. 155

socialising. 7

spousal carers. 91

staff behaviours. 11, 13

stigma. 109–10, 129

strong ties. 113

superteams. 137–38, 144, 150, 223, 228–29, 235

task-orientated care. 121

technologies, use of. 120

terminologies. 17, 19

tinnitus. 52, 78–80; challenges for health professionals. 84; and family and carers. 81–82; impacts of. 80–82; management of. 82–84; prevalence of. 79; resources. 84–85; risk factors for. 80

touch messages, developing. 204, 210, 231, 232, see also social-haptic communication

trust. 55

United Nations. 110

United Nations Convention on the Rights of Persons with Disabilities (UNCRPD). 110

unpredictable people. 54

unpredictable places. 56

unpredictable privacy. 55–56

unpredictable things. 56

unpredictable trust. 55

unrecognised/unacknowledged DSI. 32–33

Usher syndrome. 23, 47

veterans. 33–34

Vision Australia. 117

vision loss. 64; causation of. 28, 67; prevalence of. 27

visual hallucinations. 52, 60–63, 145–46, 228, see also Charles Bonnet syndrome; hallucinations

vulnerability. 37–38

weak ties. 113

we-stress. 114, 115

World Federation of the Deafblind. 20, 123–24

World Health Organisation (WHO). 110

www.ingramcontent.com/pod-product-compliance
Lightning Source LLC
Chambersburg PA
CBHW061238220326
41599CB00028B/5463